CONTENTS

D0705686

Introduction

CHAPTER 1

History of Pharmacy

Matching

Match the term to the definition.

_____ 1. dosage form

_____ 2. pharmacy shop

_____ 3. formulary

_____ 4. pharmaceutical care

A. A document that specifies particular drug forms and compositions

B. The makeup of a particular type of drug; the form in which it was given

C. Term used to describe the first stand-alone pharmacies

D. Term used to describe the care provided to a patient by the pharmacy, which encompasses all aspects of drug therapy, from dispensing to drug monitoring

Match the legislation with its description.

_____ 1. 1906 Food and Drug Act

_____ 2. 1972 Drug Listing Act

_____ 3. 1938 Federal Food, Drug, and Cosmetic Act

_____ 4. 1994 Dietary Supplement Health and Education Act

_____ 5. 1952 Durham-Humphrey Amendment

_____ 6. 1970 Comprehensive Drug Abuse Prevention and Control Act

_____ 7. 1962 Kefauver-Harris Amendment

A. Regulated claims made on the labels of herbal and dietary supplements

B. Required drugs to be safe and efficacious

C. Pharmaceuticals had to comply with their stated strengths, purity, and quality

D. Pharmaceutical products had to be safe for human use

E. Required every manufacturer or distributor of pharmaceuticals to register with the FDA, with each drug being assigned an NDC number

F. Created five drug "schedules"

G. Regulated the refilling of prescription drugs

WORKBOOK TO ACCOMPANY

The Pharmacy Technician:
A Comprehensive Approach
2nd Edition

Jahangir Moini, MD, MPH, CPhT

Professor and Former Director, Allied Health Sciences,
including the Pharmacy Technician Program
Everest University
Melbourne, Florida

Written by

Marvin L. Walker, Jr., CPhT, RPht, AAS

DAC, Supervisor, Pharmacy
CRDAMC Fort Hood, Texas

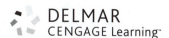

DELMAR
CENGAGE Learning™

Australia • Brazil • Japan • Korea • Mexico • Singapore • Spain • United Kingdom • United States

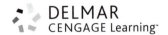

The Pharmacy Technician: A Comprehensive Approach, Second Edition
Jahangir Moini and Marvin L. Walker

Vice President, Career and Professional Editorial: Dave Garza

Director of Learning Solutions: Matthew Kane

Acquisitions Editor: Tari Broderick

Managing Editor: Marah Bellegarde

Senior Product Manager: Darcy M. Scelsi

Editorial Assistant: Ian Lewis

Vice President, Career and Professional Marketing: Jennifer Ann Baker

Marketing Manager: Kristen McNary

Marketing Coordinator: Erika Ropitsky

Production Director: Carolyn Miller

Production Manager: Andrew Crouth

Content Project Manager: Allyson Bozeth

Art Director: Jack Pendleton

Technology Project Manager: Patti Allen

Production Technology Analyst: Mary Colleen Liburdi

For product information and technology assistance, contact us at
Cengage Learning Customer & Sales Support, 1-800-354-9706

For permission to use material from this text or product,
submit all requests online at **www.cengage.com/permissions**
Further permissions questions can be emailed to
permissionrequest@cengage.com

Library of Congress Control Number: 2009936220

ISBN-13: 978-1-4354-9940-9

ISBN-10: 1-4354-9940-9

Delmar
Executive Woods
5 Maxwell Drive
Clifton Park, NY 12065
USA

Cengage Learning is a leading provider of customized learning solutions with office locations around the globe, including Singapore, the United Kingdom, Australia, Mexico, Brazil, and Japan. Locate your local office at **www.cengage.com/global**

Cengage Learning products are represented in Canada by Nelson Education, Ltd.

To learn more about Delmar, visit **www.cengage.com/delmar**

Purchase any of our products at your local bookstore or at our preferred on-line store **www.cengagebrain.com**

Notice to the Reader

Publisher does not warrant or guarantee any of the products described herein or perform any independent analysis in connection with any of the product information contained herein. Publisher does not assume, and expressly disclaims, any obligation to obtain and include information other than that provided to it by the manufacturer. The reader is expressly warned to consider and adopt all safety precautions that might be indicated by the activities described herein and to avoid all potential hazards. By following the instructions contained herein, the reader willingly assumes all risks in connection with such instructions. The publisher makes no representations or warranties of any kind, including but not limited to, the warranties of fitness for particular purpose or merchantability, nor are any such representations implied with respect to the material set forth herein, and the publisher takes no responsibility with respect to such material. The publisher shall not be liable for any special, consequential, or exemplary damages resulting, in whole or part, from the readers' use of, or reliance upon, this material.

Printed in the United States of America
3 4 5 6 7 16 15 14 13

True/False

Indicate whether the statement is true or false. If false, rewrite the statement to make it true.

_____ 1. Leaves, mud, and cool water were used to stop bleeding and heal wounds.

_____

_____ 2. Mithridates studied the adverse effects of plants and later became known as the "father of toxicology."

_____

_____ 3. The "father of medicine" was Dioscorides.

_____

_____ 4. *Aromatarii* means dealers in spices.

_____

_____ 5. There was once a belief, in 1875, that bad spirits caused diseases and that the cure for disease was to drive off the bad spirit from the sick person.

_____

_____ 6. William Proctor introduced "time management" into the practice of pharmacy in America.

_____

_____ 7. Thomas Jefferson started the first hospital in America.

_____

_____ 8. Some believe that the "Oath of Hippocrates" was written after the death of Hippocrates.

_____

_____ 9. Pharmacy is an old and intriguing profession that was once filled with mystery and unknown methods.

_____

_____ 10. The field of pharmacy has been around for only a few years.

_____

_____ 11. Dosage form refers to the route of entry into the body.

_____

_____ 12. The evolution of the profession of pharmacy can be divided into five historical periods.

_____

_____ 13. Theophrastus is the "father of botany."

_____

_____ 14. At some point in history, it was believed that only bitter medicines were efficacious.

_____

_____ 15. The Renaissance period was a time of rebirth of interest in the classical world, art, literature, philosophy, education, religion, and science.

_____

Short Answer

1. List the three major advances that occurred in pharmacy after the fall of the Roman Empire.

_____

_____

_____

_____

2. List the natural resources ancient man had to choose from when wanting to heal the sick.

_____

_____

_____

_____

3. How have the roles of pharmacists changed over the years?

_____

_____

_____

_____

4. What new scientific discoveries occurred during the Industrialization Era?

_____

_____

_____

_____

_____

CHAPTER 2

The Foundation of Pharmaceutical Care

Matching

Match the term with the definition.

_____ 1. pharmacist

_____ 2. pharmacy technician

_____ 3. profession

_____ 4. pharmacy

_____ 5. assay and control

A. Person who dispenses and counsels patients

B. A group that requires specialized education and intellectual knowledge

C. The art and science of dispensing and preparing medications and providing drug-related information to the public

D. Person who assists the pharmacist by filling prescriptions and performing other nonjudgmental tasks

E. A group with the responsibility for auditing the control system and evaluating product quality.

Match the abbreviation with its full title.

_____ 1. USP

_____ 2. NPTA

_____ 3. PTCB

_____ 4. PTCE

_____ 5. ASHP

_____ 6. AAPT

_____ 7. APhA

A. Pharmacy Technician Certification Board

B. American Association of Pharmacy Technicians

C. American Pharmacists Association

D. United States Pharmacopeia

E. Pharmacy Technician Certification Exam

F. National Pharmacy Technician Association

G. American Society of Health-System Pharmacists

True/False

Indicate whether the statement is true or false. If false, rewrite the statement to make it true.

_____ 1. In pharmaceutical care, practitioners should provide truthful, accurate, understandable information to ensure minimal patient risk and equality for all.

_____

_____ 2. The profession of pharmacy focuses on ensuring that patients receive generic drugs all the time.

_____

_____ 3. One of the characteristics of a profession is a specialized body of knowledge.

_____

_____ 4. Pharmacists have little more than a high school education.

_____

_____ 5. Pharmacy technicians assist licensed pharmacists by completing tasks that do not require the professional judgment of a pharmacist to ensure accuracy.

_____

_____ 6. PTCB stands for Pharmacy Technician Certification Board.

_____

_____ 7. Once a pharmacy technician obtains the proper licensing, no further education is required.

_____

_____ 8. A pharmacy technician may counsel patients.

_____

_____ 9. Continuing education credits can be obtained through many sources, but must be geared toward the pharmacy technician.

_____

_____ 10. Control of quality is essential in the formulation, manufacturing, and distribution of pharmaceutical products.

_____

_____ 11. A code of ethics serves to encourage respect and fair treatment for all patients.

_____

_____ 12. Like the profession of medicine, pharmacy practice has become much more specialized during the past 25 years.

_____

Short Answer

1. List five roles of a pharmacist.

_____

_____

_____

_____

_____

2. How does a pharmacy technician assist the pharmacist?

_____

_____

_____

_____

_____

3. List the three general areas of basic functional competency that the PTCB assesses.

_____

_____

_____

_____

_____

4. What is drug control and why is it important?

_____

_____

_____

_____

_____

5. List and describe five professional organizations in regard to pharmacy.

_____

_____

_____

_____

_____

_____

Multiple Choice

_____ 1. The PTCB exam is a standardized national exam for certification to become a

A. pharmacist.   C. phlebotomist.
B. pharmacy technician.   D. nurse.

_____ 2. The _____ is a nonprofit organization that sets standards for the identity, strength, quality, purity, packaging, and labeling of drug products.

A. National Pharmacy Technician Association   C. United States Pharmacopeia
B. Pharmacy Technician Educators Council   D. All of the above

_____ 3. A profession is characterized by

A. provision of a unique service to society.
B. a code of ethics.
C. a specialized body of knowledge based on advanced education, which continues to expand throughout a person's career.
D. all the above

_____ 4. According to the AACP, a Pharm D degree requires _____ years of undergraduate study followed by 4 years of graduate study.

A. 2

B. 3

C. 4

D. 5

_____ 5. The role of the pharmacy technician has been expanding in recent years, and the number of pharmacy technicians has

A. decreased.

B. increased.

C. stayed the same.

D. been unable to determine a change.

_____ 6. The skills of the pharmacy technician measured by the PTCB exam are

A. assisting the pharmacist in serving patients.

B. maintaining medication and inventory control systems.

C. participating in the administration and management of the pharmacy.

D. all the above

_____ 7. To become eligible for recertification every 2 years, certified pharmacy technicians must meet the requirements of obtaining _____ contact hours of pharmacy-related continuing education. At least _____ contact hours must be in pharmacy law.

A. 10, 2

B. 20, 1

C. 25, 1

D. 30, 2

_____ 8. The association that established a Code of Ethics for Pharmacy Technicians was

A. AAPT.

B. AAPS.

C. ACCP.

D. There is no code of ethics for pharmacy technicians.

CHAPTER 3

Pharmacy Law and Ethics for Technicians

Matching

Match the term with the definition.

_____ 1. ethics

_____ 2. law

_____ 3. misbranding

_____ 4. orphan drug

_____ 5. judicial law

_____ 6. crime

_____ 7. felony

_____ 8. misdemeanor

_____ 9. bioethics

_____ 10. national formulary

_____ 11. NDC

A. A drug that is developed for small populations of people in need of the drug

B. Rules and regulations resulting from court decisions

C. The branch of philosophy that deals with the distinction between right and wrong and with the moral consequences of human actions

D. A principle or rule that is advisable or obligatory to observe

E. Fraudulent labeling or marking

F. A less serious crime, punishable by a fine or imprisonment for less than 1 year

G. A violation of the law

H. A serious crime, such as murder, kidnapping, assault, or rape, that is punishable by imprisonment for more than one year

I. A database of officially recognized drug names

J. A discipline dealing with the ethical and moral implications of formulary biological research and applications

K. A unique and permanent product code assigned to each new drug as it becomes available in the marketplace; it identifies the manufacturer or distributor, the drug formulation, and the size and type of its packaging

Match the legislation with its description.

_____ 1. Federal Food, Drug, and Cosmetic Act of 1938

_____ 2. Durham-Humphrey Amendment of 1951

_____ 3. Poison Prevention Packaging Act of 1970

_____ 4. Controlled Substance Act of 1970

_____ 5. Drug Listing Act of 1972

_____ 6. Kefauver-Harris Amendment of 1962

_____ 7. Omnibus Budget Reconciliation Act of 1990

_____ 8. Anabolic Steroids Control Act of 1990

_____ 9. HIPAA – Health Insurance Portability and Accountability Act

_____ 10. OSHA – Occupational Safety and Health Administration

A. Created the National Drug Code

B. Established five classes of narcotics

C. This act created FDA

D. Created prescription requirements

E. Reflects an essential change of direction for drug abuse control

F. Requires that legend drugs must be in child-resistant containers

G. Requires pharmacists to offer to counsel patients

H. Requires that drug products, both prescription and nonprescription, must be effective and safe

I. Pertains to a patient's right to privacy

J. Pertains to safety in the workplace

True/False

Indicate whether the statement is true or false. If false, rewrite the statement to make it true.

_____ 1. Civil law governs the relationship between individuals within society.

_____

_____ 2. Judicial law results from actions by the legislator, whereas statutes result from court decisions.

_____

_____ 3. The mission of the DEA is to enforce controlled substances laws and regulations and to prosecute both individuals and organizations who grow, manufacture, or distribute illegal substances.

_____

_____ 4. Ethics concerns the thoughts, judgments, and actions about issues that have the greater implications of moral right and wrong.

_____

_____ 5. The FDA oversees all domestic and imported food, bottled water, and wine beverages with less than 25% alcohol.

_____

_____ 6. The FDA is a branch of the U.S. Department of Health and Human Services.

_____

_____ 7. The Omnibus Reconciliation Act of 1990 (OBRA '90) requires pharmacists to offer to discuss information about new and refilled prescriptions with Medicare and Medicaid recipients.

_____

_____ 8. The National Drug Code is used as a way to price a new drug.

_____ 9. OSHA stands for Occasionally Suspicious Handling Act.

_____ 10. Nuclear pharmacy is probably the first specialty area in the pharmacy profession for which a special regulation at the state level has been established.

_____ 11. A prescription for a controlled substance must be issued by a practitioner for a valid medical purpose.

_____ 12. The Poison Prevention Packaging Act of 1970 requires that child-resistant containers cannot be opened by 80% of children younger than age 5, but can be opened by 90% of adults.

_____ 13. If a controlled substance is lost in a pharmacy, the DEA does not need to be notified until 30 days have passed.

_____ 14. DEA form #222 is used to destroy controlled substances.

_____ 15. Any record that includes controlled substances must be made available for inspection by DEA officials.

_____ 16. DEA form #106 is used to report a controlled substance that is stolen or lost from a pharmacy.

_____ 17. When ordering controlled substances, there is not a maximum number of different items that may be ordered on the DEA form.

_____ 18. An "exempt narcotic" is an over-the-counter medication that contains only small amounts of narcotics, and therefore may be sold without a prescription, though the purchaser must be over 18 years of age and must sign a document indicating that they have received these drugs.

_____ 19. Schedule II drugs have no potential for abuse.

_____ 20. Schedule I drugs have no medical use.

_____ 21. The Comprehensive Drug Abuse Prevention and Control Act of 1970 established the five schedules used to classify controlled substances.

_____ 22. The Pure Food and Drug Act of 1906 included cosmetics.

_____ 23. Labeling was first regulated by the Sherley Amendment to the Pure Food and Drug Act of 1906.

_____ 24. Pharmacy laws of different states are different, but they are based on the same principles, objectives, and goals of pharmaceutical practice.

_____ 25. Abuse is the improper use of equipment, a substance, or a service.

_____ 26. Slander is defamatory writing.

_____ 27. Libel is spoken words that jeopardize someone's reputation or means of livelihood.

_____ 28. Fraud is dishonest and deceitful practices undertaken to induce someone to part with something of value or legal right.

_____ 29. Violations of pharmacy laws are punishable by fines or by the revocation or suspension of a license to practice.

_____ 30. As society grows and changes, laws change to conform to current realities and to try to govern future realities.

Short Answer

1. Discuss drug recall classes.

2. What is the importance of the Combat Methamphetamine Epidemic Act of 2005? What are the regulations set in place to prevent illegal use?

3. List five matters that may be discussed in counseling by a pharmacist under OBRA '90.

4. What are three examples of common OSHA violations?

_____

_____

_____

_____

_____

5. Discuss the differences between the legislative, executive, and judicial branches of the U.S. government.

_____

_____

_____

_____

_____

Multiple Choice

_____ 1. The laws relevant to the practice of pharmacy may come from different sources. An example is:

A. USDA.

B. MSDS.

C. FDA.

D. NAACP.

_____ 2. Civil law governs pharmacists who do not act in a professional manner with their customers, including areas such as

A. libel.

B. slander.

C. violation of privacy.

D. unintentional bodily injury.

E. all the above

_____ 3. Ethics are based on

A. morals.

B. law.

C. word of mouth.

D. all the above

_____ 4. The FDA regulates all drugs with the exception of

A. caplets.

B. illegal drugs.

C. capsules.

D. all the above

_____ 5. Regulatory agencies are government-based departments that create specific rules about what is and is not _____ within a specific field or area of expertise.

A. fair

B. legal

C. acceptable

D. tolerable

_____ 6. Violations against the government or the state are governed by

A. criminal law.

B. State jurisdiction.

C. pharmacy law.

D. all the above

_____ 7. _____ is considered the most serious type of crime against the government.

A. Fraud

B. Forgery

C. Treason

D. DWI

_____ 8. The failure to use a reasonable amount of care to prevent injury or damage to another is:

A. abuse.

B. fraud.

C. libel.

D. negligence.

_____ 9. Pharmacy laws of different states are different, but they are based on the same

    A. principles.   C. goals of pharmaceutical practice.

    B. objectives.   D. all the above

_____ 10. _____ agents have a high potential for abuse, but they are currently accepted for medical use in the United States.

    A. Schedule I   C. Schedule III

    B. Schedule II   D. Schedule IV

_____ 11. _____ agents have the lowest abuse potential of the controlled substances and consist of preparations containing limited quantities of certain narcotic drugs

    A. Schedule I   C. Schedule IV

    B. Schedule III   D. Schedule V

General Knowledge for the Pharmacy Technician

CHAPTER 4

Pharmaceutical and Medical Terminology and Abbreviations

Matching

Match the term with the definition.

_____ 1. prefix

_____ 2. suffix

_____ 3. abbreviations

_____ 4. chemical name

_____ 5. combining form

_____ 6. brand name

_____ 7. generic name

_____ 8. root

_____ 9. trade name

A. Shortened forms of words

B. Drug name derived from the chemical composition of the drug

C. The name that the manufacturer uses for the drug

D. A part of a word structure that occurs before or in front of the word and modifies the meaning of the root

E. A word, symbol, or device assigned to a product by its manufacturer, registered or not registered, as a trademark of its identity

F. The main part of a word that gives the word its central meaning

G. A word ending that modifies the meaning of the root

H. A root with an added vowel (known as a combining vowel) that connects the root with the suffix or the root to another root

I. A drug name, followed by the symbol®, that indicates that the name is registered to a specific manufacturer or owner and that no one else can use it.

Match the root term to its meaning.

_____ 1. angio

_____ 2. mal

_____ 3. my

_____ 4. brady

_____ 5. cardi

_____ 6. dermat

_____ 7. gluco

_____ 8. hemo

_____ 9. hepat

_____ 10. psych

A. Liver

B. Slow

C. Blood

D. Sugar

E. Vessel

F. Bad

G. Muscle

H. Heart

I. Skin

J. Mind

Match the term with its meaning.

_____ 1. diabetes

_____ 2. estrogen

_____ 3. embolism

_____ 4. hormone

_____ 5. progesterone

_____ 6. infarction

_____ 7. testosterone

_____ 8. bradycardia

_____ 9. shock

_____ 10. angina

_____ 11. cardiac arrest

_____ 12. tachycardia

_____ 13. antigen

_____ 14. hemoglobin

_____ 15. anticoagulant

_____ 16. polycythemia

_____ 17. thrombin

_____ 18. dyspnea

_____ 19. pleurisy

_____ 20. sinusitis

_____ 21. anorexia

_____ 22. emesis

_____ 23. hepatitis

_____ 24. mastication

_____ 25. prostatitis

_____ 26. nephritis

A. Chewing

B. Vomiting

C. Inflammation of the liver

D. Inflammation of a sinus

E. Lack of appetite

F. Difficulty in breathing; shortness of breath

G. A condition of too many red blood cells

H. Inflammation of the pleura, caused by injury, infection, or a tumor

I. An agent that works against the formation of blood clots

J. A blood protein that is the iron-containing pigment of red blood cells that carries oxygen from the lungs to the tissues

K. A blood enzyme that causes clotting by forming fibrin

L. The absence of a productive heartbeat

M. A state of disruption of oxygen supply to the tissue and a return of blood to the heart

N. An invading foreign substance that induces the formation of antibodies

O. Obstruction of a blood vessel by a plug (embolus)

P. Dead tissue caused by a sudden interruption of blood flow to an area; it is a term most commonly used in the context of myocardial infarction (heart attack) or cerebral infarction (stroke).

Q. Abnormally fast heartbeat; a rate of more than 100 beats per minute

R. A painful constriction or feeling of "tightness" somewhere in the body; angina pectoris is severe chest pain due to lack of oxygen and blood supply to the heart muscle.

S. A slower than normal heart rate; a rate of less than 60 beats per minute

T. A hormone produced by the corpus luteum of the ovary, the adrenal cortex, or the placenta; it is released during the second half of the menstrual cycle.

U. A hormone produced by the testes; male sex hormone

V. A chemical substance produced by the endocrine glands

W. A term describing a group of hormones produced by the ovaries; the female sex hormones

X. A general term used to describe diseases characterized by excessive discharge of urine; it is detected by the presence of large amounts of sugar in the blood due to abnormal insulin production by the pancreas.

Y. Inflammation of a kidney

Z. Inflammation of the prostate

True/False

Indicate whether the statement is true or false. If false, rewrite the statement to make it true.

_____ 1. *-cyte* is a suffix meaning "cell."

_____

_____ 2. *-dipsia* is a suffix meaning "thirst."

_____

_____ 3. *-itis* is a suffix meaning "pain."

_____

_____ 4. A prefix is a word ending that modifies the meaning of the root.

_____

_____ 5. *Auto-* is a prefix meaning "self."

_____

_____ 6. *Micro-* is a prefix meaning "large."

_____

_____ 7. *Macro-* is a prefix meaning "small."

_____

_____ 8. When a medical term is formed from two or more roots, it is called a compound word.

_____

_____ 9. Occasionally, when a prefix ends in a vowel and the root begins with a vowel, the final vowel is dropped from the prefix.

_____

_____ 10. A callus is a localized thickening of the upper skin layer due to repetitive friction.

_____

_____ 11. Hives are a fungal skin condition caused by dermatophytes or similar fungi.

_____

_____ 12. Pruritus is severe itching.

_____

_____ 13. Purpura is a yellowing of the skin due to injury.

_____

_____ 14. Ankylosis is a condition of a stiffening of a joint.

_____

_____ 15. Lumbodynia is pain in the lower back.

_____

_____ 16. The nervous system coordinates all body activities.

_____

_____ 17. The special senses of the sensory system include sight, hearing, taste, and smell.

_____

_____ 18. The eyes detect light and send signals along the optic nerve to the brain, interpreting color, shape, and dimension.

_____ 19. Pharmacy technicians must be able to communicate precisely with other professionals and specialists in different fields of health care.

_____ 20. Medical terminology, abbreviations, and symbols are not important to pharmacy technicians.

Multiple Choice

_____ 1. Most pharmacy terms have three components:

A. first, second, and third.
B. alpha, beta, and delta.

C. root, suffix, and prefix.
D. none of the above

_____ 2. The root typically identifies the

A. body part, disease, disorder, or color.
B. size and function.

C. insurance source.
D. blood type.

_____ 3. The root word Adipo means

A. male.
B. female.

C. fat.
D. gland.

_____ 4. An electrocardiogram is defined as

A. a measure of brain activity.
B. a written record of the electrical impulses of the heart.
C. a graph used by the billing department.
D. none of the above

_____ 5. The three basic types of muscle tissue are

A. skeletal.
B. smooth.

C. cardiac.
D. all the above

_____ 6. A pain in the lower back is defined as

A. arthritis.
B. collagen.

C. flatfoot.
D. lumbodynia.

_____ 7. The ears serve not only as organs of hearing but also of _____

A. balance.
B. clairvoyance.

C. beauty.
D. all the above

CHAPTER 5

Dosage Forms and Routes of Administration

Matching

Match the term with the definition.

_____ 1. ampule

_____ 2. buccal

_____ 3. caplet

_____ 4. capsule

_____ 5. elixir

_____ 6. emulsion

_____ 7. gelcap

_____ 8. induration

_____ 9. lotion

_____ 10. mixture

_____ 11. parenteral

_____ 12. powder

_____ 13. solution

_____ 14. sublingual

A. A solid dosage form in which the drug is enclosed in either a hard or soft shell of soluble material

B. An oil-based medication that is enclosed in a soft gelatin capsule

C. A small glass or plastic bottle intended to hold medicine

D. A sealed glass container that usually contains a single dose of medicine. The top must be broken off to open the container.

E. Pertaining to the inside of the cheek

F. A solid dosage form containing medicinal substances with or without suitable diluents

G. A clear, sweetened, hydroalcoholic liquid intended for oral use

H. An excessive hardening or firmness of any body site. It is one of the signs of inflammation.

I. A tablet shaped like a capsule

J. A semisolid preparation applied externally to protect the skin or to treat a dermatologic disorder

K. A mutual incorporation of two or more substances, without chemical union, in which the physical characteristics of each of the components are retained.

L. Administration by some means other than through the gastrointestinal tract

M. A system containing two liquids that cannot be mixed together in which one is dispersed, in the form of very small globules, throughout the other

N. A dry mass of minute separate particles of any substance

_____ 15. suspension

O. A liquid dosage form in which active ingredients are dissolved in a liquid vehicle

_____ 16. sustained release

P. A capsule with a controlled release of the dosage over a special period of time

_____ 17. tablet

Q. Pertaining to the area under the tongue

_____ 18. tincture

R. A liquid dosage form that contains solid drug particles floating in a liquid medium

_____ 19. topical

S. A method of intramuscular injection of medication in which the skin must be pulled to one side before the tissue is grasped for the injection of such medication. It is used when a drug is highly irritating to subcutaneous tissues or has the ability to permanently stain the skin.

_____ 20. vial

T. Pertaining to a drug that is applied to the surface of the body

_____ 21. Z-track method

U. An alcoholic solution prepared from vegetable materials or from chemical substances.

True/False

Indicate if the statement is true or false. If false, rewrite the statement to make it true.

_____ 1. A single drug may have up to three names: chemical, generic, and trade.

_____

_____ 2. Properly registered trade names become the legal property of their owners, are protected by copyright laws, and cannot be used freely in the public domain.

_____

_____ 3. New drugs may not come from living organisms, only from nonliving materials.

_____

_____ 4. Plant sources are grouped by their physical and chemical properties.

_____

_____ 5. All drugs are soluble in water.

_____

_____ 6. Most tablets are intended to be chewed for dissolution and absorption from the gastrointestinal tract.

_____

_____ 7. Buccal tablets are inserted rectally.

_____

_____ 8. Liquids may be placed in soft gelatin capsules, such as vitamin E and cod liver oil capsules.

_____

_____ 9. A small pill, usually accompanied by many others encased within a gelatin capsule, is called a granule.

_____

_____ 10. A hard or semisolid dosage form containing a medication intended for local application in the mouth or throat is called a paste or suppository.

_____

_____ 11. Bullfrog and naftifine are examples of gels.

_____

_____ 12. Transdermal patches are medicated adhesive patches placed on the skin that deliver the medication into the bloodstream directly through the skin.

_____

_____ 13. Liquid preparations do not include drugs that have been dissolved or suspended.

_____

_____ 14. A drug dosage form that consists of a high concentration of a sugar in water is called a syrup.

_____

_____ 15. Spirits are an alcohol-containing liquid that may be used pharmaceutically as a solvent.

_____

_____ 16. The nicotine transdermal patch was never used in the United States.

_____

_____ 17. Fluidextracts are not intended to be administered directly to a patient.

_____

_____ 18. In pharmacy, a mixture of distilled water with an aromatic volatile oil is called an aromatic water.

_____

_____ 19. The oral route is the safest and most convenient route chosen for most medications.

_____

_____ 20. The chosen route of drug administration does not determine the rate and intensity of the drug's effect.

_____

_____ 21. The larger the gauge of a needle is, the smaller is the diameter of its lumen.

_____

_____ 22. Always recap a needle.

_____

_____ 23. Pumps are electronic devices that force a precisely measured amount of intravenous fluid into a patient's vein over a predetermined amount of time.

_____

_____ 24. Medications that are administered through inhalers include bronchodilators, mucolytic agents, and steroids.

_____

_____ 25. Drops and ointments instilled into the eye are generally absorbed slowly and affect only the area in contact.

_____

_____ 26. Chemical names are usually applied to compounds of known composition.

_____

_____ 27. Parenteral medications never come in vials, ampules, and prefilled syringes.

_____

_____ 28. Localized infection or inflammation of the ear is treated by dropping a small amount of a sterile medicated solution into the ear.

Short Answer

1. What is the difference between disposable syringes and nondisposable syringes?

_____

_____

_____

_____

_____

2. What is the difference between intradermal, intramuscular, intravenous, and subcutaneous injections?

_____

_____

_____

_____

_____

3. In what type of infusion is a cardiovascular catheter required if it is needed for two or three days?

_____

_____

_____

_____

_____

4. What is inhalation therapy?

_____

_____

_____

_____

_____

5. List five routes of administration.

_____

_____

_____

_____

_____

Multiple Choice

_____ 1. A single drug may have up to three names:

    A. common, proper, and formal.
    B. chemical, generic, and trade.
    C. domain, copyright, and nonproprietary.
    D. manufacturer, marketable, and simple.

_____ 2. Sources of drugs include

    A. plants.
    B. animals.
    C. minerals.
    D. synthetic.
    E. all the above

_____ 3. _____ is used to prevent severe rheumatoid arthritis.

    A. Silver
    B. Mercury
    C. Gold
    D. Coal tar

_____ 4. Digoxin is made from digitalis, a derivative of the:

    A. foxglove plant.
    B. clove plant.
    C. licorice plant.
    D. carnation.

_____ 5. The newest area of drug origin is

    A. pharmacy law.
    B. gene splicing.
    C. genetic engineering.
    D. both B and C

_____ 6. The route for administering a medication depends on its

    A. form.
    B. properties.
    C. effects desired.
    D. all the above

_____ 7. _____ are commonly used for antacids and antiflatulents and for children who cannot swallow medication.

    A. Chewable tablets
    B. Gum paste
    C. Buffered caplets
    D. Flavored water

_____ 8. Buffered tablets can prevent ulceration or severe irritation of the

    A. small intestine.
    B. large intestine.
    C. stomach wall.
    D. tongue.

_____ 9. A bullet-shaped dosage form intended to be inserted into a body orifice is called a

    A. lozenge.
    B. suppository.
    C. paste.
    D. tablets.

_____ 10. An example of a transdermal patch is

    A. estrogen.
    B. fentanyl.
    C. lidocaine.
    D. all the above

_____ 11. A drug dosage form that consists of a high concentration of a sugar in water is

    A. lotion.
    B. syrup.
    C. ointment.
    D. liniment.

_____ 12. An example of a suspension is

    A. milk of magnesia.
    B. camphor.
    C. nitroglycerin.
    D. chloroform.

_____ 13. Three methods of administration are

    A. clinical, administrative, and bi polar.
    B. oral, parenteral, and topical.
    C. both A and B
    D. none of the above

_____ 14. Two types of needles are

A. disposable and nondisposable.

B. large and small.

C. nuclear and nonnuclear.

D. none of the above

_____ 15. Needle gauges range in size from

A. 5 to 10 G.

B. 16 to 35 G.

C. 13 to 31 G.

D. 14 to 40 G.

CHAPTER 6

Overview of Body Systems and Their Functions

Matching

Match the term with its definition.

_____ 1. loop of henle

_____ 2. melanin

_____ 3. sebaceous gland

_____ 4. alveolar sacs

_____ 5. arthritis

_____ 6. bursa

_____ 7. cornea

_____ 8. diaphragm

_____ 9. external acoustic meatus

_____ 10. hormones

_____ 11. insulin

_____ 12. neuron

_____ 13. osteoporosis

_____ 14. taste buds

_____ 15. venae cavae

A. Basic cell of the nervous system; carries nerve impulses

B. A dark pigment that provides skin color and absorbs ultraviolet radiation in sunlight

C. Disease that causes a reduction of bone mass

D. The portion of the nephron in the kidney that contains the tubular fluid filtered through the glomerulus

E. A system of fluid passages in the inner ear, including the semicircular canals and the cochlea

F. Skin glands that secrete an oily substance called "sebum"

G. Capillaries in the digestive system that transport fats to venous circulation

H. A U-shaped structure in the proximal convoluted tubule of the kidney; its main function is to reabsorb water and ions from the urine.

I. A hormone that extensively affects metabolism and many other body systems; it is secreted when the bold glucose level rises.

J. Natural chemical substances secreted into the bloodstream from the endocrine glands; they regulate and control organ and tissue activity.

K. The transparent front part of the eye covering the iris, pupil, and anterior chambers; it helps the eye to focus.

L. The inner skin layer, which is thicker than the epidermis

M. An important hormone involved in carbohydrate metabolism; it is antagonistic to insulin.

N. The cluster-like air sacs located at the end of each alveolar duct in the lungs

O. The study of the structure of the body

_____ 16. anatomy

_____ 17. glucagon

_____ 18. corpus callosum

_____ 19. auditory tube

_____ 20. lacteal

_____ 21. renal tubule

_____ 22. dermis

_____ 23. labyrinth

_____ 24. subcutaneous layer

P. Degenerative disease of the joints

Q. An S-shaped tube in each ear that leads inward through the temporal bone

R. The eustachian tube; the structure linking the pharynx to the middle ear

S. Capsule surrounding a joint

T. A structure in the longitudinal fissure of the brain that connects the left and right cerebral hemispheres

U. A sheet of muscle extending across the bottom part of the ribcage; it is important in the process of respiration.

V. Small structures on the upper surfaces of the tongue, soft palate, and epiglottis; they control the sense of taste.

W. The collective name for the superior and inferior vena cava, which are the veins that return deoxygenated blood from the body into the right atrium of the heart

X. A loose connective tissue layer beneath the dermis that binds the skin to underlying organs; it is predominantly made up of adipose tissue.

True/False

Indicate if the statement is true or false. If false, rewrite the statement to make it true.

_____ 1. Physiology concerns the functions of body parts—how they work and what they accomplish.

_____

_____ 2. The skin is the largest organ in the body by surface area.

_____

_____ 3. The skin forms a barrier between the inner body and the outside environment.

_____

_____ 4. Keratinocytes assist the digestive system.

_____

_____ 5. For people who have difficulty swallowing or digesting pills, transdermal patches offer an effective alternative to oral medications.

_____

_____ 6. Muscles do not require electrical impulses from motor nerves for stimulation.

_____

_____ 7. Bones of the skeletal system differ in size and shape, but are similar in structures, development, and functions.

_____

_____ 8. The skeleton is divided into two major portions: an axial skeleton and an appendicular skeleton.

_____

_____ 9. Bones are classified by shape: long, short, flat, irregular, or round.

_____

_____ 10. Joints allow the body to be mobile and flexible.

_____

_____ 11. The brainstem consists of the midbrain, pons, and medulla oblongata.

_____

_____ 12. A neuron consists of three parts: dendrites, cell body, and axons.

_____

_____ 13. The nervous system is unable to cope with different types of stressors at different times of life.

_____

_____ 14. The eye is a hollow, spherical structure about 1.2 centimeters in diameter.

_____

_____ 15. The cornea is called the "window" of the eye.

_____

_____ 16. The most common causes of blindness, worldwide, are loss of transparency of the cornea and glaucoma.

_____

_____ 17. Frequent or prolonged exposure to sounds with intensities above 185 decibels can damage the hearing receptors and cause permanent hearing loss.

_____

_____ 18. The parts of the labyrinth include three semicircular canals, which provide a sense of equilibrium, and a cochlea, which functions in hearing.

_____

_____ 19. The endocrine system consists of specialized cell clusters, glands, hormones, and target tissues.

_____

_____ 20. Endocrine glands do not secrete hormones, or chemical messengers, directly into the bloodstream.

_____

_____ 21. Most glandular activity is controlled by the pituitary gland, which is sometimes called the master gland.

_____

_____ 22. The pituitary itself is controlled by the hypothalamus.

_____

_____ 23. The hypothalamus is the main integrative center for the endocrine and autonomic nervous systems.

_____

_____ 24. The hypothalamus gland is under the control of the pituitary gland in the brain.

_____

_____ 25. Hypofunction of the posterior pituitary gland results in diabetes insipidus.

_____

_____ 26. Oxytocin produces powerful contractions of the pregnant uterus and causes milk to flow from lactating breasts.

_____

_____ 27. The thyroid gland is located in the anterior neck and is the largest of the endocrine glands.

_____ 28. The adrenal glands are located at the bottom of each kidney.

_____ 29. The conversion of glycogen to glucose results in a decrease in blood glucose.

_____ 30. If diabetes is untreated or uncontrolled, it leads to hyperglycemia.

_____ 31. Three main classes of steroid hormones are produced by gonadal tissues: estrogenic, progestational, and androgenic.

_____ 32. The most important androgenic hormone produced by the testes in men is testosterone.

_____ 33. Natural estrogenic hormones are produced by the ovaries and placenta.

_____ 34. The cardiovascular system consists of the heart and blood vessels.

_____ 35. The wall of the heart has three layers: epicardium, myocardium, and endocardium.

_____ 36. Blood consists of red blood cells, white blood cells, and platelets suspended in a liquid known as lacteals.

_____ 37. Newborns can develop physiologic jaundice a few days after birth.

_____ 38. Jaundice is an accumulation of bilirubin that turns the skin and eyes a yellowish color.

_____ 39. Platelets do not help to close breaks in blood vessels.

_____ 40. Chemical digestion is the chemical alteration of food via digestive enzymes, acids, and bile.

_____ 41. Mechanical digestion is the breakdown of large food particles into smaller pieces by chewing and the mashing actions of muscles in the digestive tract.

_____ 42. Physiology is the study of abnormal functions of the body.

_____ 43. The liver is one of the smallest organs of the digestive system.

_____ 44. Humans cannot survive without a liver.

_____ 45. The average adult liver is the heaviest organ in the body, weighing about 3 pounds.

Short Answer

1. Name the two sections of the nervous system and define them.

2. Discuss drug abuse and its addiction.

3. What is the difference between the peripheral nervous system and the autonomic nervous system?

4. Discuss the importance of the negative feedback mechanism in relationship to glandular activity.

5. List the three ways hormones are generally used in medicine.

6. What are the six hormones secreted by the anterior pituitary gland?

_____

_____

_____

_____

_____

Multiple Choice

_____ 1. Skin cells help to produce _____, which is vital for normal bone and tooth development.

    A. vitamin E   C. vitamin D

    B. vitamin A   D. vitamin K

_____ 2. The organs of the skeletal system are

    A. bones.   C. soft tissues.

    B. muscles.   D. none of the above

_____ 3. Muscles produce

    A. movement.   C. stabilize joints.

    B. maintain body posture.   D. all the above

_____ 4. The number of bones in the human body is

    A. 200.   C. 210.

    B. 206.   D. 220.

_____ 5. The brain is subdivided into the

    A. cerebrum.   D. cerebellum.

    B. diencephalon.   E. all the above

    C. brainstem.

_____ 6. The chronic self-administration of a drug in doses high enough to cause addiction is

    A. drug abuse.   C. dependence.

    B. tolerance.   D. all the above

_____ 7. The most common causes of blindness, worldwide, are loss of transparency of the cornea and

    A. glaucoma.   C. anorexia.

    B. angina pectoris.   D. vertigo.

_____ 8. Frequent or prolonged exposure to sounds with intensities above _____ decibels can damage the hearing receptors and cause permanent hearing loss.

    A. 75   C. 85

    B. 80   D. 90

_____ 9. The pituitary gland is sometimes called the

    A. first gland.   C. master gland.

    B. primary gland.   D. none of the above

_____ 10. _____ produces powerful contractions of the pregnant uterus and causes milk to flow from lactating breasts

    A. Corticosteroids   C. Rabeprazole

    B. Oxytocin   D. Omeprazole

_____ 11. Up to _____ iodine in the body is in the thyroid gland.

A. 80

B. 85

C. 90

D. 95

_____ 12. The main classes of steroid hormones are produced by gonadal tissues are

A. estrogenic.

B. progestational.

C. androgenic.

D. all the above

CHAPTER 7

Most Common Diseases and Conditions

Matching

Match the term with its definition.

_____ 1. allergens

A. Nonparasitic antigens that can stimulate a hypersensitivity reaction in certain individuals; common examples include dust, pollen, and pet dander.

_____ 2. cancer

B. The monthly flow of blood and cellular debris from the uterus; it begins at puberty and stops at menopause.

_____ 3. conjunctivitis

C. Extremely high temperature that is considered a medical emergency

_____ 4. diverticulum

D. An abnormal increase in arterial blood pressure

_____ 5. dysuria

E. The abnormal underdevelopment of the body that occurs during childhood commonly because of hyposecretion of growth hormone

_____ 6. Graves' disease

F. Malignant tumor of bottom-layer skin cells, which may also affect the eyes or bowels

_____ 7. hyperpyrexia

G. The presence of toxins in the blood

_____ 8. hypertension

H. An illness accompanying renal failure involving urinary waste products contained in the blood

_____ 9. macular degeneration

I. An inflammation of the outermost layer of the eye and inner surface of the eyelid, usually due to an allergic reaction or an infection; commonly called "pink eye"

_____ 10. melanoma

J. A condition primarily affecting older adults, wherein the macula area of the retina of the eye becomes thinner and atrophies; it often results in loss of vision.

_____ 11. menses

K. A condition of primary hyperthyroidism; it is characterized by a diffuse goiter and exophthalmos homeostasis.

_____ 12. orchitis

L. A painful condition of the testicles that may involve inflammation, swelling, and infection

_____ 13. uremia

M. The spiral shaped organ of the inner ear that contains auditory "hair cells" which provide the sense of hearing

_____ 14. toxemia

_____ 15. organ of Corti

_____ 16. peritonitis

_____ 17. dwarfism

_____ 18. emphysema

_____ 19. HDL

_____ 20. LDL

N. Inflammation of the peritoneum

O. Painful or difficult urination, often with a burning or stinging sensation

P. A group of more than 100 diseases characterized by damage to DNA, which causes abnormal cell growth and development

Q. A hollow or fluid sac, many of which exist in the walls of the colon

R. A chronic pulmonary disease characterized by loss of elasticity of the lung tissue often caused by exposure to toxic chemicals and cigarette smoke

S. Low-density lipoproteins

T. High-density lipoproteins

Match the term to its definition.

_____ 1. tinnitus

_____ 2. vertigo

_____ 3. Meniere's disease

_____ 4. GERD

_____ 5. peptic ulcers

_____ 6. nonviral hepatitis

_____ 7. viral hepatitis

_____ 8. joints

_____ 9. rheumatoid arthritis

_____ 10. PID

_____ 11. hyperpituitarism

_____ 12. cushing's syndrome

_____ 13. BPH

_____ 14. seborrheic dermatitis

_____ 15. herpes zoster

A. "Ringing in the ears"

B. Gastroesophageal reflux disease

C. A type of dizziness wherein the patient experiences the sensation of spinning or swaying while the body is actually stationary

D. Disease that affects balance and hearing, and is centered in the inner ear

E. Lesions in the mucosal membrane, which can develop in the lower esophagus, stomach, or duodenum

F. A common infection of the liver, resulting in hepatic cell destruction and necrosis

G. An inflammation of the liver that usually results from exposure to certain chemicals or drugs

H. Sites where two or more bones meet

I. A systemic inflammatory disease that attacks joints by producing inflammation of the synovial membranes that leads to the destruction of the articular cartilage and underlying bone

J. A condition of chronic hypersecretion of cortisol from the adrenal cortex, which results in excessive circulating cortisol levels

K. A chronic and progressive disease that is caused by excessive production and secretion of pituitary hormones

L. Pelvic inflammatory disease.

M. Benign prostatic hyperplasia

N. A common skin condition characterized by itchy, reddened, and oily patches of skin

O. An infection caused by the varicella-zoster virus, which is the same virus that causes chicken pox

True/False

Indicate whether the statement is true or false. If false, rewrite the statement to make it true.

_____ 1. Diseases are often described as acute or chronic.

_____

_____ 2. In the United States, cancer causes more than 300,000 deaths every year.

_____

_____ 3. Metastatic tumors develop from cancer cells that travel from an original site to a second, more distant site.

_____

_____ 4. Infection is the invasion and growth of microorganisms in or on body tissue that produces signs and symptoms of disease, as well as an immune response.

_____

_____ 5. Tendonitis is the most common causes of death in the United States.

_____

_____ 6. Angina pectoris is an episodic, reversible oxygen insufficiency.

_____

_____ 7. Myocardial infarction is also known as a heart attack.

_____

_____ 8. Ischemia is the restriction in blood supply resulting in reduced supply of oxygen.

_____

_____ 9. The peritoneum is the membrane lining parts of the abdominal cavity and visceral organs.

_____

_____ 10. The risk of hypertension decreases with age, and is lower in African Americans than Caucasians.

_____

_____ 11. Arrhythmias increase the efficiency of the heart's pumping cycle.

_____

_____ 12. Congestive heart failure is one of the most common cardiovascular disorders.

_____

_____ 13. Dietary or drug therapy of elevated plasma cholesterol levels can reduce the risk of atherosclerosis and subsequent cardiovascular disease.

_____

_____ 14. Folic acid deficiency anemia is a common, slowly progressive condition.

_____

_____ 15. Pernicious anemia is characterized by increased production of hydrochloric acid in the stomach, and an increased intrinsic factor.

_____

_____ 16. Thrombophlebitis is a deficiency in circulating blood.

_____

_____ 17. Thrombocytopenia is defined as an inflammation inside a vein along with the formation of a blood clot at the site.

_____ 18. Asthma is a respiratory condition characterized by difficulty exhaling and by wheezing.

_____ 19. Chronic bronchitis is inflammation of the bronchi caused by antibiotics.

_____ 20. A pulmonary embolism is caused by a blood clot or fat deposit formed in a peripheral blood vessel that breaks free from its site of formation and lodges in a blood vessel in the lung. This process is called thromboembolism.

_____ 21. Immunodeficiency diseases occur when the immune system is compromised and cannot react to pathogens normally.

_____ 22. People with acquired immunodeficiency syndrome are at risk of fungal and protozoal infections and skin cancers that are not usually seen in people with intact immune systems.

_____ 23. Allergic rhinitis is a reaction to airborne allergens. They are inhaled.

_____ 24. Anaphylaxis is a chronic non-life-threatening type 1 hypersensitivity reaction.

_____ 25. Latex allergy is a hypersensitivity reaction to products that contain natural latex, which is derived from the sap of the rubber tree. Latex allergy may not be affected by synthetic latex.

_____ 26. Schizophrenia and bipolar disorders are the same when it comes to diagnosis and treatment.

_____ 27. Depression is classified as a mood disorder.

_____ 28. Without proper treatment, anorexia nervosa may be fatal.

_____ 29. Dementia is a chronic deterioration of intellectual function and other cognitive skills severe enough to interfere with the ability to perform activities of daily living.

_____ 30. Anxiety disorders may be classified as generalized anxiety disorder, panic disorder, obsessive-compulsive disorder, social anxiety disorder, or posttraumatic stress disorder.

_____ 31. Panic disorder is characterized by recurrent, intensely uncomfortable episodes known as panic attacks.

_____ 32. An obsession is defined as a recurrent, persistent thought, impulse, or mental image that is unwanted and distressing, and comes involuntarily to mind despite attempts to ignore or suppress it.

_____ 33. Social anxieties are characterized by a strong desire to be with large groups of people.

_____

_____ 34. Insomnia is the ability to fall asleep and stay asleep for long periods of time.

_____

_____ 35. Alzheimer's disease has been demonstrated to be one of the most common causes of severe cognitive dysfunction in older persons.

_____

_____ 36. Seizures are classified into two basic categories: generalized and partial.

_____

_____ 37. The most common disorders of vision are age-related macular degeneration, cataracts, and glaucoma.

_____

_____ 38. The development of a cataract is usually fast, causing vision loss and possible blindness if untreated.

_____

_____ 39. Glaucoma describes a group of diseases affecting the optic nerve.

_____

_____ 40. Otitis externa is also known as swimmer's ear.

_____

_____ 41. Crohn's disease is a inflammation of the brainstem.

_____

_____ 42. Ulcerative colitis occurs primarily in the elderly, especially men.

_____

_____ 43. Falls are the most common causes of injury in people 65 years and older, with fractures of the hip and proximal humerus.

_____

_____ 44. The causes of rheumatoid arthritis have been well established and are relatively easy to treat.

_____

_____ 45. Gout often affects a single joint, such as the big toe.

_____

_____ 46. The two primary forms of diabetes mellitus are type 1 (juvenile onset) and type 2 (adult onset).

_____

_____ 47. Gonorrhea is not a sexually transmitted disease.

_____

_____ 48. Genital herpes is caused by herpes simplex virus type 2 and is a recurrent, incurable viral disease.

_____

_____ 49. Pharmacy technicians must have enough knowledge about common diseases to understand appropriate treatments.

_____

_____ 50. Cancer is the second most common disease in the United States.

_____

Short Answer

1. What is the difference between acute and chronic symptoms?

   _____

   _____

   _____

   _____

   _____

2. What is the difference between basal cell carcinoma and squamous cell carcinoma?

   _____

   _____

   _____

   _____

   _____

3. List three disorders of the central nervous system and define them.

   _____

   _____

   _____

   _____

   _____

4. What are the characteristics of Parkinson's disease?

   _____

   _____

   _____

   _____

   _____

5. What is the leading cause of blindness for people over age 50 in the United States?

   _____

   _____

   _____

   _____

   _____

6. List and describe the five major forms of hepatitis.

   _____

   _____

   _____

   _____

   _____

Multiple Choice

_____ 1. Common allergens include

    A. dust.   C. pet dander.
    B. pollen.   D. all the above

_____ 2. An inflammation of the outermost layer of the eye and inner surface of the eyelid, usually due to an allergic reaction or an infection; commonly called _____

    A. pink eye.   C. ischemia.
    B. Graves' disease.   D. necrosis.

_____ 3. In the United States, cancer causes more than _____ deaths every year, second only to cardiovascular disease.

    A. 100,000   C. 500,000
    B. 250,000   D. 100,000,000

_____ 4. There are several types of angina including

    A. stable (classic).   D. silent.
    B. unstable.   E. all the above
    C. decubitus (nocturnal).

_____ 5. Hypertension affects _____ of adults in the United States.

    A. 10% to 15%   C. 20% to 25%
    B. 15% to 20%   D. 25% to 30%

_____ 6. The risk of hypertension is higher in

    A. African Americans.   C. Native Americans.
    B. Caucasians.   D. The risk is the same for all people.

_____ 7. Each year, about _____ people in the United States experience myocardial infarction.

    A. 600,000   C. 800,000
    B. 700,000   D. 900,000

_____ 8. Common causes of pulmonary embolisms include

    A. extended confinement or bed rest.   D. trauma, injury, burns, and obesity.
    B. prolonged travel.   E. all the above
    C. recent surgery.

_____ 9. Allergic rhinitis is the most common atopic allergic reaction and affects more than _____ people in the United States.

    A. 10 million   C. 30 million
    B. 20 million   D. 40 million

_____ 10. Schizophrenia usually occurs between ages _____ in women.

    A. 15 and 25   C. 35 and 42
    B. 25 and 35   D. 45 and 48

_____ 11. Psychological components of anxiety disorders can be characterized with terms such as

    A. fear.   C. uneasiness.
    B. apprehension.   D. all the above

_____ 12. Generalized anxiety disorders may last for _____ or longer.

    A. 1 month   C. 6 months
    B. 3 months   D. 1 year

_____ 13. Proper intake of _____ can reduce the risk of developing this condition.

    A. beta-carotene   C. vitamins C and E
    B. zinc   D. all the above

Microbiology

Matching

Match the term to the definition.

_____ 1. fungi

_____ 2. Gram stain

_____ 3. antibiotics

_____ 4. coccobacili

_____ 5. agent

_____ 6. diplococci

_____ 7. antisepsis

_____ 8. autoclave

_____ 9. cocci

_____ 10. bactericidal

_____ 11. reservoir

_____ 12. portal of exit

_____ 13. fomites

_____ 14. filtration

_____ 15. pathogenic

_____ 16. portal of entry

A. A sequential procedure involving crystal violet and iodine solutions followed by alcohol that allows rapid identification of organisms as Gram-positive or Gram-negative types

B. The place where an agent can survive

C. The route by which an infectious agent leaves the reservoir to be transferred to a susceptible host

D. Microorganisms that grow in single cells or in colonies

E. Substances that have the ability to destroy or interfere with the development of a living organism

F. Short, oval-shaped bacilli

G. A chamber for sterilizing by using steam under pressure

H. An entity capable of causing disease

I. Able to destroy bacteria

J. Spherical bacteria that occur in pairs

K. Capable of producing disease

L. The route by which an infectious agent enters the host

M. Microorganisms that stain blue or purple with Gram stain

N. Agents, such as microorganisms, that cause disease

O. Substances that destroy most microorganisms, but not highly resistant types such as certain spores and viruses

P. A process of cleaning that destroys most microorganisms, but not highly resistant types such as certain spores and viruses

____ 17. pathogens

Q. The process of passing a substance through a filter to remove specific particles

____ 18. fungicidal

R. Related to physiology as well as chemistry

____ 19. disinfectant

S. A process of converting organic compounds, such as carbohydrates, to simpler compounds, such as ethyl alcohol, by using enzymes that do not require oxygen; fermentation usually results in the production of energy.

____ 20. microorganisms

T. Objects contaminated with an infectious agent but are symptom free

____ 21. disinfection

U. Having a killing action on fungi

____ 22. spirilla

V. Organisms that are too small to be seen by the unaided eye

____ 23. spores

W. Preventing infection by arresting or inhibiting growth and multiplication of infectious agents

____ 24. staphylococci

X. Spherical or semispherical bacteria

____ 25. streptococci

Y. Spiral-shaped bacteria, or other types of microorganisms, that require oxygen to survive

____ 26. sterilization

Z. The study of symptoms of diseases

____ 27. sporicidal

AA. A resistant stage of bacteria that can withstand an unfavorable environment

____ 28. symptomatology

BB. A substance that kills spores

____ 29. virions

CC. Round or oval-shaped, Gram-positive bacteria occurring in pairs or chains

____ 30. Gram-positive

DD. The procedure of destroying all microorganisms in order to prevent the spread of infection

____ 31. physiochemical

EE. Spherical, Gram-positive, and parasitic bacteria usually occurring in grape-like clusters

____ 32. fermentation

FF. Complete RNA or DNA particles surrounded by protein shells that constitute infectious forms of viruses

True/False

Indicate if the statement is true or false. If false, rewrite the statement to make it true.

____ 1. The importance of microorganisms cannot be overemphasized.

_____

____ 2. Microbiology is defined as the study of organisms and agents too small to be seen clearly by the unaided eye.

_____

____ 3. Spores are resistant to heat, drying, and disinfectants.

_____

_____ 4. Viruses are organisms that can live only outside cells.

_____ 5. Bacteria are classified into two groups based on their capacity to be stained.

_____ 6. Rickettsia are small bacteria capable of living free of a host.

_____ 7. Without the transmission of microorganisms, the infectious process cannot occur.

_____ 8. Transmission by touching is the most common means of transmitting pathogens.

_____ 9. An example of vehicle transmission is spores of anthrax.

_____ 10. A compromised host is a person whose normal defense mechanisms are impaired and who is therefore more susceptible to infection.

_____ 11. The single most important means of preventing the spread of infection is frequent and effective hand hygiene by all health care workers.

_____ 12. Proper hand washing depends on two factors: running water and age.

_____ 13. There are no microorganisms that are beneficial.

_____ 14. Pharmacy technicians must focus on the control of microorganisms by physical, chemical, and biological agents.

_____ 15. A bleach solution is an effective disinfectant for surfaces that have come into contact with viruses, including HIV.

_____ 16. Small instruments may be sufficiently disinfected by soaking them in 70% to 80% isopropanol alcohol for 10 to 25 minutes.

_____ 17. Antisepsis is the prevention of infection or sepsis by using antiseptics.

_____ 18. Antiseptics are just as toxic as disinfectants.

_____ 19. Trichomonas vaginalis is a common protozoal infection.

Multiple Choice

_____ 1. The most effective method for destruction of all types of microorganisms is:

A. filtration.
B. HEPA filters.

C. autoclave.
D. gas sterilization.

_____ 2. Green pigments found in plants and other photosynthetic organisms.

A. Bacilli
B. Chlorophyll

C. Cocci
D. Diplococci

_____ 3. Viral infections include:

A. colds.
B. hepatitis.

C. genital herpes.
D. all of the above.

_____ 4. Contact with an infected person through contaminated secretions is called:

A. contact transmission.
B. airborne transmission.

C. vehicle transmission.
D. vector-borne transmission.

_____ 5. A person experiencing a compromised emotional state has lower defense mechanisms. This is called:

A. lifestyle.
B. heredity.

C. stress.
D. concurrent disease.

_____ 6. Characteristics of viruses include:

A. They can live only inside cells.
B. They contain a core of DNA or RNA surrounded by a protein coating.
C. Some can create an additional coating called an envelope that protects it from attack by the immune system.
D. All of the above.

_____ 7. Pathogenic bacteria cause a wide range of illnesses, including:

A. diarrhea.
B. pneumonia.

C. sinusitis.
D. all of the above.

Short Answer

1. What are some ways of preventing diseases that people can practice?

_____

_____

_____

_____

_____

2. Discuss the three types of agents capable of causing disease.

_____

_____

_____

_____

_____

3. Discuss what is meant by "the chain of infection."

_____

_____

_____

_____

_____

4. What are the "links" in this chain?

_____

_____

_____

_____

_____

CHAPTER 9

Pharmacology

Matching

Match the term to its definition.

_____ 1. anxiety

_____ 2. antihistamines

_____ 3. bactericidal

_____ 4. bronchodilators

_____ 5. seizure

_____ 6. sedatives

_____ 7. opioids

_____ 8. opiates

_____ 9. hypnotic

_____ 10. hypnosis

_____ 11. hormones

_____ 12. metered-dose inhaler

_____ 13. cation

A. Narcotic alkaloids found in opium

B. Drugs that block neuromuscular transmission at the neuromuscular junction; they cause paralysis of specific skeletal muscles.

C. A temporary, abnormal electrical brain condition that results in abnormal neuronal activity; it can affect mental ability and cause convulsions.

D. A handheld pressurized device used to deliver medications for inhalation

E. A drug that induces sleep; often used to treat insomnia and in surgical anesthesia

F. A trance-like state that resembles sleep that is induced by the suggestions of one person upon another who accepts them as effective

G. A positively charged atom

H. Also known as "spasmolytics," these agents alleviate musculoskeletal pain and spasms to reduce spasticity

I. An intense, involuntary muscle contraction or spasm, as is commonly seen during a seizure condition

J. The most potent and consistently effective anti-inflammatory agents that are currently available for relief of respiratory conditions

K. Chemical substances that have morphine-like action in the body; commonly used for pain relief

L. A degenerative disorder of the central nervous system that usually impairs motor skills, speech, and other functions

M. The use of a sedative agent to reduce excitement, nervousness, or irritation; commonly prior to a medical procedure

_____ 14. hypertension

_____ 15. sedation

_____ 16. hyperlipidemia

_____ 17. convulsion

_____ 18. corticosteroids

_____ 19. antitussive

_____ 20. angina pectoris

_____ 21. arrhythmias

_____ 22. antibiotics

_____ 23. bacteriostatic

_____ 24. Parkinson's disease

_____ 25. neuromuscular blocking agents

_____ 26. dry powder inhaler

_____ 27. centrally acting skeletal muscle relaxants

N. Substances that suppress the central nervous system, and induce calmness, relaxation, drowsiness, or sleep

O. Condition that describes chest pain, lack of blood and oxygen supply to the heart muscle, usually because of vessel obstruction or spasm

P. Therapeutic agents that slow or stop the growth of microorganisms

Q. Drugs that counteract the action of histamine

R. A physiological state consisting of fear, apprehension, or worry

S. Agents that relax the smooth muscle of the bronchial tubes

T. Capable of killing bacteria. This term is typically used in reference to antiseptics, disinfections, or antibiotics.

U. Various conditions of abnormal electrical heart activity; the heart may beat too fast, too slow, or irregularly.

V. A drug that reduces coughing, also called a "cough suppressant"

W. Capable of stopping the growth and reproduction of bacteria

X. A device used to deliver medication in the form of micronized powder into the lungs

Y. Chemical messengers that move through the blood or through cells that carry signals

Z. The presence of raised or abnormal levels of lipids or lipoproteins in the blood

AA. High blood pressure.

True/False

Indicate whether the statement is true or false. If false, rewrite the statement to make it true.

_____ 1. Examples of hormones include melatonin, epinephrine, dopamine, and insulin.

_____

_____ 2. Hypertension is a chronic elevation of the blood pressure equivalent to or greater than 140/90.

_____

_____ 3. Pharmacy technicians do not need to have a wide understanding of the types of drugs available, or their uses.

_____

_____ 4. Clinical pharmacology is the study of the biologic effects of a drug on a patient when it is used as a medical treatment.

_____

_____ 5. Parkinson's disease has no visible physical characteristics.

_____

_____ 6. Depression is the second most common psychiatric disorder in the United States.

_____

_____ 7. Psychosis is characterized by hallucinations and delusions.

_____

_____ 8. Endocrine drugs are used to treat deficiencies or excesses of specific hormones, or nonendocrine diseases.

_____

_____ 9. Regular insulin can only be administered intravenously.

_____

_____ 10. Medications are the first line of treatment for hyperlipidemia.

_____

_____ 11. Clot formation is vital to prevent bleeding from cuts and other injuries.

_____

_____ 12. Anticoagulants are agents that prevent formation of blood clots.

_____

_____ 13. Some of the most common disorders in humans at any age are those affecting the digestive system.

_____

_____ 14. Barbiturates have a higher risk of adverse effects and toxicity than benzodiazepines.

_____

_____ 15. Insulin dosage is measured in milligrams.

_____

_____ 16. Penicillins were one of the first antibiotics developed.

_____

_____ 17. Penicillin allergies can be fatal.

_____

_____ 18. Sulfonamides were the first drugs to prevent and cure human bacterial infections successfully.

_____

_____ 19. Vancomycin can destroy most Gram-negative organisms.

_____

_____ 20. Patients taking metronidazole are warned about the dangerous effects of drinking alcohol while taking the drug.

_____

_____ 21. HAART involves the combination of three to four drugs that are effective against HIV.

_____

_____ 22. The primary lesion of tuberculosis is located in the lungs.

_____

_____ 23. Diarrhea is the manifestation of many illnesses.

_____

_____ 24. Nonopioid antidiarrheals are the most effective drugs for controlling diarrhea.

_____

_____ 25. Fluoxetine is the generic name for Prozac.

_____

Multiple Choice

_____ 1. Narcotic analgesics are:

A. referred to as opioids.
B. not used for pain management.
C. used only to treat gout.
D. not legal in any form.

_____ 2. Hypertension:

A. may go untreated with little bodily harm.
B. does not lead to heart attacks or strokes.
C. is treated by using diuretics, beta-blockers, calcium channel blockers, as well as other drugs.
D. is not dangerous.

_____ 3. Heart arrhythmias occur because of:

A. improper impulse generation.
B. improper conduction.
C. A and B.
D. none of the above.

_____ 4. Invading microorganisms include:

A. viruses.
B. bacteria.
C. fungi.
D. all the above.

_____ 5. Manipulating estrogen and progesterone levels can prevent:

A. viral infections.
B. hypertension.
C. hypotension.
D. pregnancy.

_____ 6. Semisynthetic antibiotics structurally and pharmacologically related to penicillins are:

A. macrolides.
B. cephalosporins.
C. sulfonamides.
D. tetracyclines.

_____ 7. Fluoroquinolones are related to:

A. citric acid.
B. boric acid.
C. nalidixic acid.
D. sulfuric acid.

_____ 8. DNA viruses include:

A. herpes simplex 1 and 2.
B. varicella-zoster.
C. influenza A.
D. all the above.

_____ 9. Commonly used devices for inhalation include:

A. metered-dose inhaler.
B. dry powder.
C. nebulizers.
D. all of the above.

_____ 10. Carbamazepine is the generic name for:

A. Dilantin.
B. Depakene.
C. Tegretol.
D. Valium.

Short Answer

1. What is the difference between a general anesthetic and a local anesthetic?

_____

_____

_____

_____

_____

2. Discuss the differences between the two general classifications for diabetes mellitus.

_____

_____

_____

_____

_____

3. Discuss the three groups into which penicillins are classified.

_____

_____

_____

_____

_____

4. What is "Red Man Syndrome"?

_____

_____

_____

_____

_____

5. List three generic and brand names that are examples of anesthetics.

_____

_____

_____

_____

_____

6. Discuss the different onset of action times for the four types of insulin discussed in this chapter.

_____

_____

_____

_____

_____

CHAPTER 10

Immunology and Vaccines

Matching

Match the term with its definition.

_____ 1. active acquired immunity

_____ 2. allergen

_____ 3. allergy

_____ 4. anthrax

_____ 5. antibodies

_____ 6. antigens

_____ 7. antitoxin

_____ 8. attenuation

_____ 9. B lymphocytes

_____ 10. contraindication

_____ 11. diphtheria

_____ 12. erythema migrans

_____ 13. *Haemophilus influenzae*

A. A zoonotic disease caused by the anthrax bacillus that can infect humans in a number of ways and can be fatal

B. Inflammation of the liver caused by microorganisms, especially viruses, or drugs such as alcohol and other poisons

C. Cells of the adaptive immune system that express cell surface immunoglobulins specific for an epitope on an antigen

D. Proteins that develop in response to the presence of antigen in the body and react with the antigen on the next exposure. Antibodies may be formed from infections, immunization, transfer from mother to child, or unknown antigen stimulation.

E. The ability of a substance, such as an antigen, to provoke an immune response

F. Antibodies that neutralize toxins

G. An antigen

H. A fear of water: a symptom caused by rabies as the disease progresses

I. An acute, toxin-mediated disease by *Corynebacterium diphtheriae*

J. Immunity resulting from the development of antibodies within a person's body that renders the person immune; it may occur from exposure through a disease process or from immunizations

K. An immunologic reaction that destroys or resists antigens

L. A hypersensitive reaction to foreign substances (allergens) by the immune system

M. Foreign substance that causes the production of specific antibodies

_____ 14. hepatitis

N. A rash often seen in the early stages of Lyme disease. The rash represents an actual skin infection with Lyme bacteria.

_____ 15. hydrophobia

O. A foreign substance (such as pollen, dander, or mold) that can cause an allergic reaction in hypersensitive people

_____ 16. immunity

P. A Gram-negative bacterium that commonly causes otitis media or bacterial meningitis in children

_____ 17. immunogen

Q. A condition that increases the chance of a serious adverse reaction

_____ 18. immunogenicity

R. The process of weakening pathogens

Match the term to its definition.

_____ 1. immunoglobulins

A. Large, granular lymphocytes that appear to have the ability to destroy tumor cells

_____ 2. immunology

B. Blood products that contain disease specific antibodies for passive immunity

_____ 3. inactivated vaccines

C. An acute viral infectious disease

_____ 4. influenza A

D. Vaccines containing living organisms or intact viruses that have undergone radiation or temperature conditioning to produce safe vaccinations that will help the patient become immune to a specific disease

_____ 5. influenza B

E. The study of immune responses

_____ 6. influenza C

F. Immunity acquired from the injection or passage of antibodies from an immune person or animal to another for short-term immunity or immunity passed from mother to child

_____ 7. killer cells

G. An inflammation of the meninges (membranes) that surround and protect the brain. It is often caused by bacteria

_____ 8. live attenuated vaccines

H. Resistance to the causative pathogen in individuals who have had a specific infection because of the presence of antibodies and stimulated lymphocytes

_____ 9. Mantoux test

I. An acute viral illness

_____ 10. measles

J. A virus causing moderate to severe illness, affecting all age groups

_____ 11. meningitis

K. An intradermal screening for tuberculin hypersensitivity. A red, firm patch of skin at the injection site greater than 10 mm in diameter after 48 hours is a positive result that indicates current or prior exposure to tubercle bacilli.

_____ 12. mumps

L. Inflammation of the salivary glands

_____ 13. myocarditis

M. A virus causing a mild illness; usually only affects children

_____ 14. natural active acquired immunity

N. Inflammation of the heart

_____ 15. parotitis

O. A viral infection of the upper respiratory tract

_____ 16. passive acquired immunity

P. Vaccines in which the infectious components have been destroyed by chemical or physical treatments

Match the term to its definition.

_____ 1. pertussis

_____ 2. plasma cells

_____ 3. pneumonia

_____ 4. poliomyelitis

_____ 5. precaution

_____ 6. rabies

_____ 7. Reye's syndrome

_____ 8. rubella

_____ 9. smallpox

_____ 10. tetanus

_____ 11. tine test

_____ 12. T lymphocytes

_____ 13. toxoid

_____ 14. tuberculosis

_____ 15. vaccination

A. Differentiated B cells that secrete antibodies.

B. An acute inflammation of the lungs, often caused by inhaled *streptococcus pneumoniae*

C. Specific warning to consider when medications are prescribed or administered

D. Inflammation of the spinal cord that leads to paralysis

E. An acute infectious disease caused by the bacterium *Bordetella pertussis*; also known as whooping cough

F. An acute, often fatal disease caused by an exotoxin produced by *Clostridium tetani.*

G. Acute viral disease that was essentially eradicated in 1979 that causes a disfiguring rash, headache, vomiting, and fever

H. A mild, highly infectious viral disease common in childhood

I. A complication that occurs almost exclusively in children taking aspirin, primarily in association with influenza B or varicella zoster, and presents with severe vomiting and confusion, which may progress to coma, due to swelling of the brain

J. The only rhabdovirus that infects humans; it is a zoonotic disease characterized by fatal meningoencephalitis.

K. In this test, the tuberculin antigen is infected just under the skin with a multipronged instrument. The antigen is located on the spikes that penetrate the skin. If results are positive, the skin around the injection site will be red and swollen like a mosquito bite 48 to 72 hours after the injection.

L. A chronic granulomatous infection caused by *Mycobacterium tuberculosis*. It is generally transmitted by the inhalation or ingestion of injected droplets and usually affects the lungs.

M. A toxin that has been treated with chemicals or heat to decrease its toxic effect but retain its antigenic powers

N. Lymphocytes that exhibit cell surface receptors that recognize specific antigenic peptide-major histocompatibility complexes.

O. The process of immunization for prevention of diseases

True/False

Indicate if the statement is true or false. If false, rewrite the statement to make it true.

_____ 1. Most infections in normal individuals are short-lived and leave little permanent damage.

_____

_____ 2. The site of the infection and the type of pathogen largely determine which immune responses will be effective.

_____

_____ 3. A person who is susceptible to a disease usually has an adequate level of protective antibodies or sufficient nonspecific defenses.

_____

_____ 4. Vaccines are made from living or dead pathogens or from certain toxins they excrete.

_____

_____ 5. Vaccines made from dead organisms are the most effective.

_____

_____ 6. Another word for allergy is *hypersensitivity.*

_____

_____ 7. Pharmacists are never allowed to administer selected immunizations, such as flu vaccines, in retail pharmacies.

_____

_____ 8. Immunoglobulins must be kept refrigerated similarly to vaccines.

_____

_____ 9. Human immunoglobulins should be kept at room temperature.

_____

_____ 10. Adverse reactions do not include local or severe systemic reactions.

_____

_____ 11. Mumps is a chronic viral illness.

_____

_____ 12. Antibodies are also known as immunoglobulins.

_____

_____ 13. Pregnant women may receive the influenza vaccine by injection, but should not receive the nasal influenza spray vaccine while they are pregnant.

_____

_____ 14. Yellow fever is a viral infection transmitted by mosquitoes, commonly in countries outside of the United States.

_____

_____ 15. Anthrax was first used effectively as a bioterrorist agent in 1900.

_____

Multiple Choice

_____ 1. The immune system protects the body initially by creating:

A. local barriers.
B. inflammation.
C. more red blood cells.
D. both A and B.

_____ 2. The normal concentration of IgG in the blood is about:

    A. 50% to 60%.   C. 90% to 100%.
    B. 70% to 80%.   D. None of the above.

_____ 3. Newborn babies do not have their own:

    A. antibodies.   C. white blood cells.
    B. red blood cells.   D. identity.

_____ 4. The incubation period of diphtheria is:

    A. 1 to 2 days.   C. 6 to 7 days.
    B. 2 to 5 days.   D. 8 to 10 days.

_____ 5. Approximately _____ of patients with measles have one or more complications.

    A. 10%   C. 30%
    B. 20%   D. 50%

_____ 6. Live attenuated virus vaccines include:

    A. measles.   C. rubella.
    B. mumps.   D. all the above.

_____ 7. Routine childhood smallpox vaccination was discontinued in the United States in:

    A. 1961.   C. 1981.
    B. 1971.   D. 1991.

Short Answer

1. Discuss the first line, second line, and third line of defense the body uses to protect itself from disease.

_____

_____

_____

_____

_____

2. Discuss the three stages of pertussis.

_____

_____

_____

_____

_____

3. Discuss the basic antigen types.

_____

_____

_____

_____

_____

4. What are the three major risk groups for hepatitis B?

_____

_____

_____

_____

_____

5. What is the difference between active and passive immunity?

_____

_____

_____

_____

_____

CHAPTER 11

Nutrition

Matching

Match the term to its definition.

_____ 1. calcium

_____ 2. biotin

_____ 3. copper

_____ 4. fats

_____ 5. ascorbic acid

_____ 6. chloride

_____ 7. electrolytes

_____ 8. cholesterol

_____ 9. calciferol

_____ 10. lipids

_____ 11. pharma food

_____ 12. fatty acids

_____ 13. fluoride

_____ 14. folic acid

_____ 15. iodine

_____ 16. iron

A. An alkali metal element that helps regulate neuromuscular excitability and muscle contraction

B. The only one of six essential nutrients containing nitrogen

C. A fat-soluble vitamin essential for skeletal growth, maintenance of normal mucosal epithelium, reproduction, and visual acuity

D. Any of several organic acids produced by the hydrolysis of neutral fats

E. Fats

F. A disease caused by extreme lack of protein

G. A common metallic element essential for the synthesis of hemoglobin

H. An essential micronutrient of the thyroid hormone

I. A water-soluble vitamin essential for cell growth and the reproduction of red blood cells

J. Any substance that becomes part of a food product

K. A substance that prevents tooth decay and protects against osteoporosis and gum disease

L. A nonmetallic chemical element occurring extensively in nature as a component of phosphate rock

M. A phosphorus-containing lipid

N. The sum of the processes involved in the taking in of nutrients and their assimilation and use for proper body functioning and maintenance of health

O. A chemical substance found in food that is necessary for good health

P. A part of two enzymes that regulate energy metabolism

_____ 17. kwashiorkor

_____ 18. food additive

_____ 19. minerals

_____ 20. niacin

_____ 21. nutrient

_____ 22. nutrition

_____ 23. phospholipid

_____ 24. phosphorus

_____ 25. menadione

_____ 26. marasmus

_____ 27. magnesium

_____ 28. protein

_____ 29. potassium

_____ 30. retinol

Q. Inorganic substances occurring naturally in the earth's crust, having a characteristic chemical composition

R. A water-soluble, injectable form of the product of vitamin K3

S. Severe wasting caused by lack of protein and all nutrients or faulty absorption

T. A silver-white mineral element; the second most abundant cation of the intracellular fluids in the body and is essential for many enzyme activities

U. A system of nourishing through breathing

V. Substances composed of lipids or fatty acids and occurring in various forms

W. Compounds that dissociate into ions when dissolved in water

X. A water-soluble vitamin that is essential for the formation of collagen and fibroid tissue for teeth, bones, cartilage, connective tissue, and skin

Y. A water-soluble B complex vitamin that acts as a coenzyme in fatty acid production and in the oxidation of fatty acids and carbohydrates

Z. A metallic element that is a component of several important enzymes in the body and is essential to good health

AA. A waxy lipid found only in animal tissues

BB. An anion of chlorine

CC. An alkaline earth metal element

DD. A fat-soluble vitamin chemically related to the steroids and essential for the normal formation of bones and teeth

True/False

Indicate if the statement is true or false. If false, rewrite the statement to make it true.

_____ 1. Carbohydrates are nutrients providing the main source energy in the average diet.

_____

_____ 2. Cyanocobalamin is a fat-soluble substance that is the common pharmaceutical form of vitamin B6.

_____

_____ 3. Feeding by tube directly into the patient's digestive tract is known as enteral nutrition.

_____

_____ 4. HDLs, LDLs, and VLDLs are basically the same term.

_____

_____ 5. Malnutrition is the ingestion of nutrients inadequate to maintain health and well-being.

_____

_____ 6. Hyperalimentation is the administration of a nutritionally adequate hypertonic solution consisting of glucose, protein, minerals, and vitamins through an indwelling catheter into the superior vena cave.

_____

_____ 7. Pantothenic acid is a member of the vitamin B complex.

_____

_____ 8. TPN stands for total parental nutrition. It is an intravenous feeding that supplies all the nutrients necessary for life.

_____

_____ 9. Sodium is one of the most unimportant elements in the body.

_____

_____ 10. One of the heat-stable components of the B complex vitamins is riboflavin.

_____

_____ 11. Vitamins are organic substances necessary for life, although they do not independently provide energy.

_____

_____ 12. Human growth and development does not require both nutritional and psychosocial support.

_____

_____ 13. Carbohydrates are the major source of building material for muscles, blood, skin, hair, nails, and the internal organs.

_____

_____ 14. The term *lipid* is used to describe both fats and oils.

_____

_____ 15. Fat-soluble include vitamins A, D, E, and K.

_____

_____ 16. Water-soluble include vitamins B and C.

_____

_____ 17. Vitamin A has essential roles in development of vision, bone growth, maintenance of epithelial tissue, the immunological process, and normal reproduction.

_____

_____ 18. Exposure to the sun for 30 minutes every day allows skin to provide enough vitamin D for the body.

_____

_____ 19. Vitamin K is stored in the body and is toxic.

_____

_____ 20. Heat and prolonged cooking, especially cooking with water, can destroy B vitamins.

_____

_____ 21. Minerals function in many metabolic roles in the body.

_____

_____ 22. Food items and supplements must be labeled in the pharmacy.

_____

_____ 23. The Nutrition Labeling and Education Act of 1990 requires that most packaged foods have a list of a specified set of nutrition facts on the label.

_____

_____ 24. No single food supplies all the nutrients needed by the body.

_____

_____ 25. Pharmacy technicians do not need to be familiar with basic nutrition dietary standards and pathological conditions.

_____

Multiple Choice

_____ 1. Neutral fats consist of what percentage of triglycerides or triacylglycerols?

A. 100%   C. 90%
B. 95%   D. 85%

_____ 2. A fat-soluble vitamin essential for normal reproduction, muscle development, resistance of erythrocytes to hemolysis, and various other biochemical functions.

A. Tocopherol   C. Vitamin B7
B. Thiamin   D. Vitamin B2

_____ 3. A water-soluble, crystalline compound of the B complex, essential for normal metabolism and health of the cardiovascular and nervous systems is:

A. sodium.   C. vitamin B1.
B. vitamin B6.   D. thiamin.

_____ 4. Simple fat compounds consisting of three molecules of fatty acid and glycerol is:

A. triglycerides.   C. pyridoxine.
B. vitamin B complex.   D. vitamin A.

_____ 5. A water-soluble vitamin that is essential for the formation of collagen and fibroid tissue for teeth, bones, cartilage, connective tissue, and skin is:

A. vitamin K.   C. vitamin C.
B. vitamin E.   D. vitamin D.

_____ 6. Vitamin K is also called:

A. calciferol.   C. tocopherol.
B. quinones.   D. ascorbic acid.

_____ 7. Life expectancy in the United States is:

A. decreasing.   C. staying unchanged.
B. increasing.   D. undetermined.

_____ 8. Good fats are known as:

A. HDL.   C. VLDL.
B. LDL.   D. phospholipids.

_____ 9. Zinc deficiency is characterized by:

A. abnormal fatigue.   C. a decrease in taste and odor sensitivity.
B. decreased alertness.   D. all the above.

_____ 10. Enteral tube feedings are contraindicated in patients with the following:

A. diffused peritonitis.   C. intractable vomiting.
B. severe diarrhea.   D. all the above.

Short Answer

1. What is the difference between hypovitaminosis and hypervitaminosis?

_____

_____

_____

_____

_____

2. What is the difference between vitamins B1, B2, B3, B6, B7, B9, and B12?

_____

_____

_____

_____

_____

3. Discuss the normal range versus abnormal range when referring to cholesterol and lipoproteins.

_____

_____

_____

_____

_____

4. What are some of the symptoms and diseases associated with mineral deficiencies?

_____

_____

_____

_____

_____

CHAPTER 12

Food and Drug Interactions

Matching

Match the term to its definition.

_____ 1. synergism

_____ 2. potentiation

_____ 3. drug interaction

_____ 4. cytochrome P-450

_____ 5. antagonism

A. A system of enzymes that contributes to drug interactions

B. The cooperative effect of two or more drugs given together to produce a stronger effect than that of either drug given alone

C. When two drugs act to decrease the effects of each other

D. An interference of a drug with the effect of another drug, nutrient, or laboratory test

E. One drug prolongs the effects of another drug

True/False

Indicate whether the statement is true or false. If false, rewrite the statement to make it true.

_____ 1. All drug-related problems develop expectedly and are usually predicted.

_____

_____ 2. Many drug-related problems are caused by drug interaction.

_____

_____ 3. Antacids can inhibit the gastric absorption of tetracycline.

_____

_____ 4. Many drugs used currently have the capacity to influence many physiological systems.

_____

_____ 5. Pharmacy technicians do not need to be aware of drug-related problems when dealing with patients.

_____

_____ 6. Physicians are always aware of all the drugs that have been prescribed by other doctors for a patient.

_____

_____ 7. Age is always an important factor in the risk of drug interaction.

_____

_____ 8. Newborn infants have fully developed enzyme systems.

_____

_____ 9. Genetic factors may be responsible for the development of an unexpected drug response in some patients.

_____

_____ 10. Food often may affect the rate and extent of absorption of drugs from the gastrointestinal tract.

_____
_____

11. Estrogen, midazolam, and all calcium channel blockers should not be taken with grapefruit juice.

_____

_____ 12. Vegetables such as broccoli, cabbage, or brussels sprouts may inactivate anticoagulants such as warfarin.

_____

_____ 13. Chronic use of alcoholic beverages may decrease the rate of metabolism of drugs such as warfarin.

_____

_____ 14. Patients should be encouraged to ask questions about their therapy.

_____

_____ 15. It is not necessary to maintain complete and current medication records for patients.

_____

_____ 16. MAO inhibitors may interact, with potentially toxic effects with wine, cheese, or yogurt.

_____

_____ 17. Medications that stimulate the central nervous system may cause a toxic stimulation if caffeine or caffeine-containing foods are also consumed.

_____

_____ 18. Simvastatin is the generic name for Zocor.

_____

_____ 19. Promethazine is the generic name for Demerol.

_____

_____ 20. Older patients who may be taking five or six medications can forget to take them.

_____

Multiple Choice

_____ 1. Surgical patients commonly receive more than:

A. 5 drugs.	C. 15 drugs.
B. 10 drugs.	D. 20 drugs.

_____ 2. When two drugs with similar actions are taken, the effect of the drugs will:

A. double.	C. cancel each other.
B. triple.	D. have no effect.

_____ 3. What agents are most often abused?

A. Opioids

B. Barbiturates

C. Analgesics

D. All the above

_____ 4. Smoking increases the activity of drug-metabolizing enzymes in the:

A. liver.

B. spleen.

C. brain.

D. small intestine.

_____ 5. The pharmacist has a valuable opportunity to make a significant contribution to further enhance the:

A. efficacy of drug therapy.

B. safety of drug therapy.

C. Both A and B

D. None of the above

Short Answer

1. Give examples of synergism, antagonism, and potentiation.

_____

_____

_____

_____

_____

2. What are the factors that influence the response to a drug in humans?

_____

_____

_____

_____

_____

3. What are four drugs that will metabolize more rapidly because of smoking?

_____

_____

_____

_____

_____

Medication Errors

Matching

Match the term to its definition.

_____ 1. biologics

_____ 2. transcription

_____ 3. trailing zeros

_____ 4. clinical

_____ 5. hematoma

_____ 6. leading zeros

_____ 7. malpractice

_____ 8. negligence

_____ 9. pain scales

A. The process of entering a physician's order into a computer

B. Zeros that follow decimal points

C. Charts used to measure a patient's pain intensity level

D. The failure to do something that a reasonable person might do, or doing something that a reasonable person might not do

E. Negligence performed by a professional, such as a pharmacist, or a pharmacist-supervised technician

F. Zeros that precede decimal points

G. A localized mass of blood outside of the blood vessels that appears to be discolored

H. Having to do with the examination and treatment of patients

I. Agents that give immunity to diseases or living organisms

True/False

Indicate whether the statement is true or false. If false, rewrite the statement to make it true.

_____ 1. A medication error is any preventable event that causes or leads to inappropriate medication use or patient harm.

_____

_____ 2. When a drug is manufactured incorrectly, including how it is packaged, a drug recall may be the result.

_____

_____ 3. Highly trained people rarely make a mistake.

_____

_____ 4. The physician's order must be clarified if it is unclear.

_____

_____ 5. Always assume that a patient is the correct person to receive a medication even without verifying his or her name.

_____

_____ 6. Dosing errors are the least common medication errors that occur in adults and children.

_____

_____ 7. Poor communication between staff members can also result in errors.

_____

_____ 8. The health care provider who has the responsibility of administering a medication has the final opportunity to avoid a mistake.

_____

_____ 9. Both internal and external noise can interrupt the concentration of health care workers and cause medication errors.

_____

_____ 10. If pharmacy technicians are not adequately supervised due to staff shortages, they may make errors that will go unchecked by pharmacists or other personnel.

_____

_____ 11. Stress is not linked to a variety of outcomes.

_____

_____ 12. Every patient's pain tolerance level is the same.

_____

_____ 13. Patients should rely on their doctors' expertise and never question their medications.

_____

_____ 14. Herbal remedies may interact dangerously with certain medications prescribed by a physician, dispensed by a pharmacist, or administered by a nurse.

_____

_____ 15. The FDA's MedWatch program encourages the voluntary reporting of adverse events or product problems.

_____

_____ 16. Pharmacists and technicians can not join an electronic mailing list to get up-to-date information that the FDA disseminates.

_____

_____ 17. A pharmacist or a supervised pharmacy technician who violates a regulation or law that establishes a standard of care that is designed to protect patients may be guilty of negligence.

_____

_____ 18. Labels should be checked and compared with physicians' orders at least five times to ensure accuracy.

_____

_____ 19. MedWatch provides important and timely clinical information about safety issues involving products.

_____

_____ 20. Upon detecting an error in dispensing, the pharmacy technician must take all necessary steps to rectify it promptly and notify the pharmacist immediately.

_____

Multiple Choice

_____ 1. The Institute for Safe Medication Practices estimates that approximately _____ Americans die each year as a result of medical errors.

A. 88,000   C. 108,000
B. 98,000   D. 118,000

_____ 2. Deaths in U.S. hospitals due to medical errors exceed _____ per year, which is more than deaths from motor vehicle accidents, breast cancer, and AIDS.

A. 22,000   C. 44,000
B. 33,000   D. 55,000

_____ 3. According to the Institute for Safe Medication Practices, which medications have the "highest alert" concerning medication errors?

A. Insulin and heparin
B. Narcotics and opiates
C. Potassium chloride injections
D. All the above

_____ 4. Fatigue has many effects that can allow medication errors to occur. They include:

A. slowed reaction times.
B. reduced accuracy.
C. inability to recognize changes in the patient.
D. all the above.

_____ 5. The term "every other day" is abbreviated:

A. AD.   C. QOD.
B. TIW.   D. IU.

_____ 6. The term "right eye" is abbreviated:

A. OD.   C. QID.
B. D/C.   D. HS.

_____ 7. Penalties concerning negligence or malpractice may include:

A. restriction on practice and fines.
B. suspension of ability to practice and jail sentences.
C. revocation of ability to practice.
D. all the above.

_____ 8. A pharmacist who fails to perform a prospective drug regimen review, gives incorrect advice, or doesn't warn a patient about potential adverse effects is guilty of:

A. slander.   C. malpractice.
B. breach of contract.   D. libel.

_____ 9. The Joint Commission requires organizations to prove that their personnel are:

A. legal U.S. citizens. C. able to read English.

B. competent. D. physically fit.

Short Answer

1. Discuss the factors that may cause administering errors.

_____

_____

_____

_____

_____

2. Discuss the essential items that the technician must keep in mind.

_____

_____

_____

_____

3. Discuss the two medication error reporting systems.

_____

_____

_____

_____

_____

Mathematics and Calculations Review

CHAPTER 14

Basic Mathematics

Matching

Match the term to its definition.

_____ 1. Arabic numbers

_____ 2. common fraction

_____ 3. complex fraction

_____ 4. decimal

_____ 5. decimal fraction

_____ 6. denominator

_____ 7. divisor

_____ 8. extremes

_____ 9. fraction

_____ 10. improper fraction

_____ 11. means

_____ 12. mixed fraction

_____ 13. multiplicand

_____ 14. multiplier

_____ 15. numerator

A. The answer to a division problem

B. A whole number and a proper fraction that are combined. The value of the mixed number is always greater than 1.

C. The answer from multiplying two or more quantities together

D. Standard numerical numbers

E. An expression of division with a number that is the portion or part of a whole

F. The portion of the whole being considered

G. A numerator that is expressed in numerals, with a decimal point placed so that it designates the value of the denominator, and the denominator, which is understood to be 10 or some power of 10; also called decimal

H. The relationship between two equal ratios

I. The number to be multiplied by another

J. The numerator or the denominator or both as a whole number, proper fraction, or mixed number. The value may be less than, greater than, or equal to 1.

K. A numerator that is expressed in numerals with a decimal point placed so that it designates the value of the denominator, and the denominator, which is understood to be 10 or some power of 10; also called decimal fraction

L. The number performing the division

M. The numerator is greater than or equal to the denominator

N. A mathematical expression that compares two numbers by division

O. Equal parts of a whole

_____ 16. percent

_____ 17. product

_____ 18. proper fraction

_____ 19. proportion

_____ 20. quotient

_____ 21. ratio

P. The two inside terms in a ratio

Q. The two outside terms in a ratio

R. The numerator is smaller than the denominator and designates less than one whole unit

S. The number the whole is divided into

T. A fraction whose numerator is expressed and whose denominator is understood to be 100

U. A number by which another is multiplied

True/False

Indicate whether the statement is true or false. If false, rewrite the statement to make it true.

_____ 1. The system of Roman numerals uses letters to represent number values.

_____ 2. Roman numerals are used more commonly than Arabic numbers in dosage calculation.

_____ 3. The metric system is the system most often used in the calculation of drug dosages.

_____ 4. In some cases, one must determine the lowest common denominator by the method of trial and error.

_____ 5. The smallest whole number that can be divided evenly by all denominators is known as the lowest common denominator.

_____ 6. When calculating drug dosages, it is helpful to know whether the value of one fraction is greater or less than the value of another fraction.

_____ 7. Technicians must be able to convert from one measurement system to another.

_____ 8. The extremes are the two outside terms, and the means are the two inside terms.

_____ 9. Correct drug dosage calculations are one of the most important factors in the prevention of medication errors.

_____ 10. Technicians are required to understand basic mathematics in order to be able to calculate drug dosages by weight, volume, and by using balances.

Problem Solving

1. An order calls for Meperidine 10mg IM q6h prn pain. Meperidine 15mg/ml is in stock. How many milliliters will the nurse administer in a 24-hour period?

2. What is the concentration of a 1 gram Vancomycin vial that is reconstituted with 20 ml of water?

3. A nurse wants to give 10 mg of betamethasone. The syringe says the concentration is 2.5mg/ml. How many mls does the nurse need for the dose?

4. Make 40 mEq of KCL in 1000 ml of normal saline. KCL concentration is 20mEq/10ml. How many mls would you need to add to the IV bag?

5. How many milliliters of a solution are needed to prepare a 150 mg dose if the concentration is 500 mg in 5 ml?

CHAPTER 15

Measurement Systems

Matching

Match the term with its definition.

_____ 1. dram

_____ 2. grain

_____ 3. gram

_____ 4. household system

_____ 5. international units

_____ 6. liter

_____ 7. meter

_____ 8. metric system

_____ 9. milliequivalent

_____ 10. milliunit

_____ 11. minim

_____ 12. ounce

_____ 13. unit

A. The basic unit for length in the metric system

B. The amount of medication required to produce a certain effect

C. A unit of weight in the apothecary system

D. The basic unit of volume in the apothecary system

E. Worldwide standard system of measurement

F. A unit of measure based upon the chemical combining power of a substance

G. One-thousandth of a unit

H. The basic unit for volume in the metric system

I. System of measurement used in most homes; this is not an accurate system of measurement for medications.

J. The basic unit for weight in the metric system

K. The basic unit of weight in the apothecary system

L. A unit of weight in the apothecary system

M. A standardized amount of medication required to produce a certain effect

True/False

Indicate which statement is true or false. If false, rewrite the statement to make it true.

_____ 1. Pharmacy technicians must have a comprehensive knowledge of the weights and measures used in drug administration for prescribed amounts.

_____

_____ 2. A kilo is equal to one thousand units.

_____

_____ 3. A liter is equal to 500 milligrams.

_____

_____ 4. 1 gr equals 60 mg or 1 gr equals 65mg.

_____

_____ 5. 1 lb equals 2.2 kg.

_____

_____ 6. 60 drops are equivalent to a teaspoon.

_____

_____ 7. Household measurements are very accurate and should be used at all times when measuring medication.

_____

_____ 8. 240 mL is equal to 16 oz.

_____

_____ 9. The apothecary system of measurement is rarely used in the clinical setting, and is one of the oldest of the various measurement systems.

_____

_____ 10. Sodium bicarbonate and potassium chloride are examples of drugs that are measured in milliequivalents.

_____

_____ 11. Pharmacy technicians must be able to convert and calculate the correct dosage of drugs.

_____

_____ 12. 3 teaspoons is equal to 4 oz.

_____

_____ 13. There are 15 teaspoons in 5 tablespoons.

_____

_____ 14. 32 oz is equal to 4 cups.

_____

_____ 15. 2000 mcg is equal to 2 mg.

_____

Multiple Choice

_____ 1. Which system is the most accurate and popular system used today for drug prescriptions and drug administration?

    A. Metric   C. Household

    B. Apothecary   D. European

_____ 2. The abbreviation for centimeter is:

    A. mcg.   C. cm.

    B. cc.   D. kg.

_____ 3. A system for international standardization of metric units was established throughout the world in:

    A. 1950.   C. 1970.

    B. 1960.   D. 1979.

_____ 4. Which one of the following drugs is ordered in units?

    A. Meclizine   C. Heparin

    B. Metronidazole   D. Oxytocin

_____ 5. To change grams to milligrams, _____ 1000 and move the decimal point three places to the right.

    A. add   C. multiply by

    B. subtract   D. divide by

Short Answer

1. What are the three systems used in measuring medication and solutions?

_____

_____

_____

_____

_____

2. How many pounds does a patient weigh if he is 98 kg?

_____

_____

_____

_____

_____

3. How many kg does a patient weigh if he is 250 lb?

_____

_____

_____

_____

_____

Unit Conversions

1. 500 mg = _____ g

2. 40 kg = _____ lb

3. 4000 mL = _____ L

4. 240 mL = _____ oz

5. _____ mg = 1000 g

6. 350 mcg = _____ mg

7. _____ mL = 45.45 L

8. 2 gr = _____ mg

9. _____ kg = 100 g

10. 600 g = _____ kg

11. _____ mL = 8 oz

12. 65 mg = _____ gr

13. 25 mg = _____ g

14. 45 cc = _____ mL

15. 1.5 g = _____ mg

16. 2.2 lb = _____ kg

17. 0.5 g = _____ mg

18. 0.5 g = _____ gr

19. 237.5 cm = _____ in

20. 8 mL = _____ L

21. 0.01 g = _____ mcg

22. 4 mg = _____ g

23. 300 g = _____ kg

24. 16 oz = _____ cups

25. _____ cups = 480 mL

26. 2 cups = _____ mL

27. _____ oz = 4 cups

28. 8 oz = _____ t

29. 2 T = _____ mL

30. 6 g = _____ kg

31. 150 lb = _____ kg

32. 6 t = _____ T

Problem Solving

1. A patient is prescribed Inderal 30 mg p.o. QID. On hand are 10 mg tablets. How many tablets must be dispensed?

2. A patient is prescribed Urcholine 50 mg, p.o., TID for 10 days. On hand are 100 mg tablets. How many tablets must be dispensed?

3. A patient is prescribed 60 mg Lasix, p.o., BID for 7 days. On hand is 40 mg tablets. How many tablets must be dispensed?

4. A patient is prescribed Tranxene 7.5 mg, p.o., q.am. On hand is 3.75 mg tablets. How many tablets must be dispensed?

Calculation of Dosages

Matching

Match the term with its definition.

_____ 1. conversion factor

_____ 2. dosage strength

_____ 3. drop rate

_____ 4. drug label factor

_____ 5. form

_____ 6. meniscus

_____ 7. nomogram

_____ 8. supply dosage

_____ 9. total volume

A. The structure and composition of a drug

B. A quick reference for calculating pediatric doses

C. Used to determine equivalents of specific units of measure

D. The quantity contained in a package

E. Refers to both the dosage strength and the form of the drug; the number of measured units per tablet of the concentration of a drug

F. The amount of medication per unit of measure

G. The number of drops an intravenous infusion is administered at over a specific period of time

H. The form of the drug dose with its equivalent in unit

I. The curved upper surface of a column of a liquid in a container

True/False

Indicate whether the statement is true or false. If false, rewrite the statement to make it true.

_____ 1. One of the most important functions of pharmacy service is to ensure that patients get the intended drug in the correct amount.

_____

_____ 2. Learning to correctly calculate drug dosages is an extremely important skill, because it can often be the difference between life and death for a patient.

_____

_____ 3. The right hospital is one of the ways to prevent medication errors.

_____

_____ 4. The NDC number tells the technician how many tablets are required to fill a prescription.

_____

_____ 5. Dosage strength of a drug refers to its dosage weight, the amount of the drug provided in a specific unit of measurement.

_____

_____ 6. The administration route refers to the site of the body or the method of drug delivery intended.

_____

_____ 7. D stands for desired dose; H stands for on-hand dose; V stands for vehicle.

_____

_____ 8. A variety of forms of drugs are commonly administered orally. These include tablets, capsules, powders, and liquids.

_____

_____ 9. When a liquid medication is measured, hold the transparent measuring device at waist level.

_____

_____ 10. After the dry form of the drug is reconstituted with sterile water, bacteriostatic water, or saline, the medication is used immediately or must be refrigerated.

_____

_____ 11. Usually, the reconstituted drug in the vial is used within 48 hours to 1 week.

_____

_____ 12. Dilantin is a potent anticoagulant that prevents clot formation and blood coagulation.

_____

_____ 13. Heparin is available in only an oral dosage.

_____

_____ 14. Maintenance fluids help patients maintain normal electrolyte and fluid balances.

_____

_____ 15. To measure the flow rate, the drip chamber must be squeezed until it is ¼ full, making it easier to appropriately count the number of drops falling into the chamber.

_____

_____ 16. Macrodrop tubing is used for slower infusions for which accuracy of dosage delivery is essential.

_____

_____ 17. A flow rate is the speed at which intravenous fluids are infused into a patient.

_____

_____ 18. Total parenteral nutrition (TPN) is also called hyperalimentation.

_____

Multiple Choice

_____ 1. A pharmacy technician must recognize the:

A. generic name.   C. dosage strength.
B. trade name.   D. all the above.

_____ 2. Certain drugs are dispensed in a powder form and must be:

    A. reconstituted.   C. sent back to the manufacturer.

    B. inhaled.   D. used only in an emergency.

_____ 3. By federal law, all medications must be identified with control numbers, sometimes called:

    A. Rx numbers.   C. lot numbers.

    B. PTCB numbers.   D. DL numbers.

_____ 4. Examples of cautions or alerts that certain drug may need are:

    A. "Refrigerate at all times."   C. "Protect from light."

    B. "Keep in a dry place."   D. All the above.

_____ 5. There are two very important reasons for identifying the unit being calculated first:

    A. It eliminates any confusion over exactly which measure is being calculated.

    B. It dictates how the first ration factor is entered in the equation.

    C. Both A and B

    D. None of the above

_____ 6. Insulin is supplied in 10 mL vials labeled with the number of units per milliliter; thus, "U-100 insulin" means there are:

    A. 10 U/mL.   C. 1000 U/mL.

    B. 100 U/mL.   D. None of the above.

Short Answer

1. List six different administration routes.

_____

_____

_____

_____

_____

2. Discuss the four methods for drug dosage calculations.

_____

_____

_____

_____

_____

3. Why are children more sensitive to medications than are adults?

_____

_____

_____

_____

4. What are the three formulas used to calculate dosage for infants and children?

_____

_____

_____

_____

_____

Problem Solving

1. A dosage of 24 mg has been ordered. The solution strength available is 12.5 mg in 1.5 mL. How many mL will be dispensed?

2. Rx is diphenhydramine HCI 25 mg p.o. BID PRN for agitation. Available is Diphenhydramine hydrochloride elixir 12.5mg/5ml. How many mL will be dispensed?

3. Rx is Haldol 10 mg p.o. BID. Available is Haldol concentrate labeled 2mg/mL. How many mL will be dispensed?

4. Rx is Tagamet 400 mg p.o q6h. Available is Tagamet labeled 300mg/5mL. How many mL will be dispensed?

5. If a patient purchases 2 pint bottles of antacid and takes 2 tablespoonfuls every 6 hours, how many days will the antacid last?

6. How many mL of an antibiotic containing 0.2 mg/mL of a drug would provide a 125-mg dose?

7. How many mL of digoxin elixir containing 50 mcg/mL would provide a 0.5-mg dose? If the normal dose of a drug is 200 mcg, how many doses can be given from a multiple dose vial containing 0.03 g of the drug?

8. If a patient takes diazepam 2 mg TID for 30 days, how many grams of diazepam will the patient receive after 30 days of therapy?

9. Rx digoxin 0.68 mg p.o. BID. On hand is digoxin 325 mcg/cc 2-oz bottle.

   • How may mL of the supply is required per ordered dose?

• How many doses are in the 2-oz supply bottle?

• How many days will the 2-oz bottle last?

• How many mcg of Lanoxin will the patient get in 7 days?

• How many mL are needed for a 30-day supply?

10. Rx Zithromax 798 mg p.o. TID for 7 days. On hand is Zithromax 100mg/tsp in 8-oz bottles.

• How many mg is ordered per dose?

• How many mL of the supply is required per dose?

• How many gm will the patient receive in 7 days?

• How many doses can the patient get out of the 8-oz stock bottle?

• How many days will the 8-oz bottle last?

• How many mL are needed to fill the order?

11. Dr. orders Amoxil 330 mg p.o. q 6 h for 10 days. Your pharmacy stocks Amoxil 250mg/tsp in 6-oz bottles.

• How many mg is ordered per dose?

• How many mL of the supply is required per dose?

- How many gm will the patient receive in 10 days?

- How many doses can the patient get out of the 6-oz stock bottle?

- How many days will the 6-oz bottle last?

- How many mL are needed to fill the order?

12. Order D5W to infuse at 100 mL/hr. Drop factor: 10gtt/mL. How many gtt/min should the I.V. be regulated at?

13. Order 1,500 mL 0.9% NS in 10 hours. Drop factor: 20 gtt/mL. How many gtt/min should the I.V. infuse at?

14. The doctor orders 100 U of regular insulin to be added to 500 mL of 0.45% saline to infuse at 10 U per hour. The I.V. flow rate should be how many mL per hour?

15. Order 15 U of regular insulin per hour. 40 U of insulin is placed in 250 mL of NS.

   • How many mL/hr should the I.V. infuse at?

   • Drop factor: 60 gtt/mL. Calculate the gtt/min.

16. An I.V. is regulated at 20 microgtt/min. How many hours will it take for 100 mL to infuse?

Pharmacy Practice Settings

Safety in the Workplace

Matching

Match the term with its definition.

_____ 1. barrier precautions

_____ 2. biohazard symbol

_____ 3. carcinogenic

_____ 4. caustic

_____ 5. ergonomic

_____ 6. exposure control plan

_____ 7. fire safety and emergency plan

_____ 8. hazard communication plan

_____ 9. material safety data sheet (MSDS)

_____ 10. universal precautions

_____ 11. teratogenic

A. A set of guidelines for infection control

B. A substance that causes developmental malformation to an embryo or fetus

C. Written or printed material concerning a hazardous chemical that includes information on the chemical's identity and physical and chemical characteristics

D. Application of warning labels for all hazardous chemicals

E. A written procedure that includes fire extinguisher locations, fire alarm pull-box locations, sprinkler system location, exit signs, and clear directions to the quickest and safest exit of a building during an emergency

F. A written procedure for the treatment of persons exposed to biohazardous or similar chemically harmful material

G. The science of designing equipment to maximize productivity by lessening the discomfort and fatigue of employees

H. A substance that eats away at something

I. A substance that causes cancer

J. Measures taken to minimize the risk of exposure to blood and body fluids

K. An image or object that serves as an alert that there is a risk to organisms, such as ionizing radiation or harmful bacteria or viruses

True/False

Indicate whether the statement is true or false. If false, rewrite the statement to make it true.

_____ 1. OSHA establishes dress code regulations for employers and monitors compliance.

_____

_____ 2. OSHA requires pharmacies to have a material safety data sheet (MSDS) for each hazardous chemical material used.

_____

_____ 3. Each MSDS contains basic information about the specific chemical or product.

_____

_____ 4. The top diamond on a hazardous label indicates hazards to health.

_____

_____ 5. Category I employees are employees who are at the greatest risk of exposure to communicable diseases via blood, body fluids, and other potentially infectious materials while at work.

_____

_____ 6. Job descriptions should identify anything that could potentially cause exposure to hazardous chemicals and bloodborne pathogens.

_____

_____ 7. About one-third of all occupational injuries reported by employers are work-related musculoskeletal disorders.

_____

_____ 8. OSHA regulations do not require that all health care workers be immunized against hepatitis B.

_____

_____ 9. Companies with more than 100 employees must maintain records of all work-related injuries and illnesses.

_____

_____ 10. When technicians prepare, compound, or dispense medications, hand washing and clean techniques are critical.

_____

_____ 11. All needles can be thrown in regular trash cans.

_____

_____ 12. Pharmacies have spill cleanup kits in areas where potentially harmful chemicals and substances are used.

_____

_____ 13. Hazardous materials include any substance that is not clean, disinfected, or sterilized, or that is corrosive, cytotoxic, ignitable, radioactive, reactive, toxic, or caustic.

_____

_____ 14. Any materials that have come into contact with blood or body fluids are treated as hazardous waste.

_____

_____ 15. Solid waste is not considered hazardous, but can pollute the environment.

_____

_____ 16. OSHA's primary concern is protection of employees from biological and chemical hazards.

_____

_____ 17. Ergonomics is also referred to as "human engineering" and "human factors."

_____

Multiple Choice

_____ 1. In what year did the federal government pass the Occupational Safety and Health Act?

A. 1960　　　　　　　　　　　　　　　　C. 1980
B. 1970　　　　　　　　　　　　　　　　D. 1990

_____ 2. In 1991, OSHA set forth the Bloodborne Pathogens Standard to improve infection control education. The standard was intended to reduce occupational cases of:

A. HIV and HBV.
B. PVC and HBV.
C. AAA and PVC.
D. CAC and HIV.

_____ 3. Approximately _____ of health care workers are sensitive to latex, and should use "latex-free" or "hypoallergenic" gloves made of either vinyl or nitrile.

A. 4% to 6%　　　　　　　　　　　　　　C. 14% to 20%
B. 8% to 12%　　　　　　　　　　　　　　D. over 25%

_____ 4. Health care workers must use appropriate personal protective equipment, such as:

A. gloves and masks.　　　　　　　　　　C. gowns and goggles.
B. lab coats and face shields.　　　　　　　D. all the above.

_____ 5. Barrier precautions include:

A. personal protective equipment.　　　　　C. proper hazardous waste containment.
B. immunizations.　　　　　　　　　　　　D. all the above.

Short Answer

1. Discuss OSHA's safety guidelines for the pharmacy technician.

_____

_____

_____

_____

_____

2. List five things that are listed on a MSDS.

_____

_____

_____

_____

_____

3. What are the three types of allergic reactions to latex?

_____

_____

_____

_____

_____

CHAPTER 18

Hospital Pharmacy Practice

Matching

Match the term with its definition.

_____ 1. automation

_____ 2. Centers for Medicare & Medicaid

_____ 3. department of health

_____ 4. controlled substance medication order

_____ 5. demand/stat medication order

_____ 6. computerized physician order entry system

_____ 7. emergency medication order

_____ 8. floor stock system

_____ 9. group purchasing

_____ 10. hospital pharmacy

_____ 11. independent purchasing

_____ 12. investigational medication order

A. An organization that surveys and accredits health care organizations

B. An order for a medication given under direction of research protocols that also require strict documentation of procurement, dispensing, and administration

C. The director of the pharmacy or buyer directly contacts and negotiates pricing with pharmaceutical manufactures

D. The provision of pharmaceutical services within an institutional or hospital setting

E. Many hospitals working together to negotiate with pharmaceutical manufacturers to get better prices and benefits based upon the ability to promise high committed volumes

F. A system of drug distribution in which drugs are issued in bulk form and stored in medication rooms on patient care units

G. The automatic control or operation of equipment, processes, or systems, and often involves robotic machinery controlled by computers

H. An organization that inspects and approves institutions to provide Medicaid and Medicare services

I. An inventory control system in which stock arrives just before it is needed

J. The written order for particular medications and services to be provided to a patient within an institutional setting

K. An order for a medication to be given in response to a medical emergency

L. An organization that oversees hospitals, including the pharmacy department

_____ 13. The Joint Commission

M. An order for medication to be given in rapid response to a specific medical condition

_____ 14. just-in-time system

N. An order for medication that requires monitored documentation of procurement, dispensing, and administration

_____ 15. medication order

O. A computerized system in which the physician inputs the dedication order directly for electronic receipt in the pharmacy

_____ 16. patient prescription system

P. A system of drug distribution in which a nurse supplies the pharmacy with a transcribed medication order for a particular patient and the pharmacy prepares a 3-day supply of the medication

_____ 17. policy

Q. A system for distributing medication in which the pharmacy prepares single doses of medications for a patient a 24-hour period

_____ 18. policies and procedures manual

R. A substance that contains no living microorganisms

_____ 19. PRN medication order

S. An agency that registers pharmacists and pharmacy technicians

_____ 20. procedure

T. An order for medication that is to be given on a continuous schedule

_____ 21. scheduled intravenous/ total parenteral nutrition solution order

U. An order for medication given via an infection; these medications are to be prepared in a controlled environment.

_____ 22. scheduled medication order

V. Statement of a series of steps to implement the policies of the department or organization

_____ 23. state board of pharmacy

W. An order for medication to be given in response to a specific defined parameter or condition

_____ 24. sterile product

X. A formal document specifying guidelines for operations of an institution

_____ 25. unit-dose drug distribution system

Y. Statement of the definite course or method of action selected to support goals of the overall organization

Match the organization with its mission.

_____ 1. Food and Drug Administration

A. Policies and procedures to show proper handling of controlled substances

_____ 2. Drug Enforcement Administration

B. Policies and procedures showing implementation of its guidelines and standards of practice

_____ 3. Occupational Safety and Health Administration

C. Investigation of drug policies and procedures in hospital pharmacies and drug recall policies and procedures

_____ 4. The Joint Commission

D. Policies and procedures that ensure the health and safety of people in the workplace

_____ 5. American Society of Health-System Pharmacists

E. Policies and procedures that guide the pharmacy department in providing safe, effective, and cost-effective drug therapy

True/False

Indicate whether the statement is true or false. If false, rewrite the statement to make it true.

_____ 1. Dispensing processes have become less sophisticated than in the past in response to the need to handle a variety of different pharmacy settings.

_____

_____ 2. Hospital pharmacies control the cost of their inventories either by purchasing directly from pharmaceutical manufacturers or by using group purchasing.

_____

_____ 3. Because of the increased elderly population and the number of new medications being introduced, the future of the hospital pharmacy looks very bright.

_____

_____ 4. The director of pharmacy is responsible for all the pharmacy services provided in or by the organization.

_____

_____ 5. The medication fulfillment process ends in the pharmacy department when a copy of the original medication order is received in the department.

_____

_____ 6. The role of the pharmacist has not changed from being a product dispenser to having expanding responsibility for the entire medication process.

_____

_____ 7. Hand washing is a very important procedure for preventing contamination.

_____

_____ 8. Customers of pharmacy services expect to have drugs quickly, cheaply, of high quality, and that have been stored properly.

_____

_____ 9. Automation has the ability to simplify narcotic drug inventory and tracking records.

_____

_____ 10. Human intervention can always be replaced.

_____

_____ 11. The increasing complexity of health care in the modern hospital is creating ever-greater demands for the hospital pharmacy to broaden its scope of services.

_____

_____ 12. It is not necessary for a pharmacy technician to utilize aseptic techniques when preparing compounded products.

_____

_____ 13. Data entry is an important part of the pharmacy technician's job.

_____

_____ 14. Ordering and maintenance of stock levels is often the responsibility of the pharmacy technician.

_____

_____ 15. Each filled medication order must be appropriately labeled with the patient's name, medical record number, room number, name of the prescriber, date of dispensing, name of the drug, the strength of the drug, quantity of the drug dispensed, dosage dispensed, dosage directions, and expiration date.

_____

_____ 16. The label does not need to have the initials of the persons dispensing the drug.

_____

_____ 17. Policies and procedures should relate to the selection, distribution, and safe and effective use of drugs in the facility.

_____

Multiple Choice

_____ 1. The personnel in a hospital pharmacy are classified into three categories. In order, from highest to lowest, they are:

A. support, professional, technical.   C. technical, support, professional.
B. professional, technical, support.   D. support, technical, professional.

_____ 2. The medication order must contain the following information:

A. dosage schedule and strength.
B. patient's name, height, weight, date of birth, medical record number, medical condition, and known allergies.
C. route of administration and direction for use.
D. instructions for preparing the drugs.
E. all the above.

_____ 3. A disadvantage of the floor stock system is:

A. decreased inventory needs.
B. no possibility of drug diversion.
C. potential for medication errors.
D. adequate space for medication storage on the patient care unit.

_____ 4. Many unit-dose systems use the _____ hour medication cart exchange process.

A. 12   C. 36
B. 24   D. 48

_____ 5. The roles and duties of the technician in the hospital setting are:

A. maintenance of medication records and compounding medications.
B. preparing unit doses and packaging.
C. computer data input and maintaining privacy.
D. working safety and communication skills.
E. all the above.

_____ 6. Pharmacy technician re-certification requires:

A. 20 continuing education credits with 1 being in pharmacy law every 2 years.
B. 30 continuing education credits with 1 being in pharmacy law every 2 years.
C. 40 continuing education credits with 1 being in pharmacy law every 2 years.
D. 50 continuing education credits with 1 being in pharmacy law every 2 years.

_____ 7. The _____ monitors the use of scheduled drugs and those who prescribe them.

A. FCC   C. FBI
B. ECC   D. DEA

_____ 8. For scheduled drugs, federal law requires records be kept on file for _____ years, depending on a state's law.

A. 1–3

B. 2–5

C. 7–9

D. 10–11

Short Answer

1. What are several types of services provided by a pharmacy within an institution?

_____

_____

_____

_____

_____

2. Discuss the organizational structure of a hospital or health care system.

_____

_____

_____

_____

_____

3. Discuss the modes of purchasing.

_____

_____

_____

_____

_____

CHAPTER 19

Community Pharmacy

Matching

Match the term with its definition.

_____ 1. drive-through

_____ 2. inscription

_____ 3. legend drug

_____ 4. over-the-counter (otc)

_____ 5. pharmacy compounding

_____ 6. professionalism

_____ 7. signa

_____ 8. subscription

_____ 9. superscription

A. Medication prescribed

B. Rx symbol

C. Dispensing directions to pharmacist

D. Directions for patient

E. The following of a profession as an occupation and conforming to the rules and standards of the profession

F. An external site at a pharmacy that can be accessed by driving up in the car

G. A medication that may be dispensed only with a prescription; also known as prescription drug

H. A medication that may be purchased without a prescription directly from the pharmacy

I. The preparation, mixing, assembling, packaging, or labeling of a drug or device

True/False

Indicate whether the statement is true or false. If false, rewrite the statement to make it true.

_____ 1. Community pharmacies are classified into two categories, independent and chain pharmacies.

_____

_____ 2. Wal-Mart is an example of a chain pharmacy.

_____

_____ 3. The pharmacist or pharmacy technician not only must be precise in the manual aspects of filling the prescription order but also must provide the patient with the necessary information and guidance to assure the patient's compliance in taking the medication properly.

_____

_____ 4. Pharmacy technicians should read the prescription completely and carefully to be sure the ingredients or quantities prescribed are clear.

_____

_____ 5. It is a legal requirement that the prescription order be numbered, but the same number does not have to be placed on the label.

_____

_____ 6. The name, address, and telephone number of the pharmacy are all legally required to appear on the label.

_____

_____ 7. Auxiliary labels are placed on prescription bottles and are used to prevent product tampering.

_____

_____ 8. It is not necessary to wipe down the counting tray after each tablet has been counted because contamination rarely occurs.

_____

_____ 9. The number of refills of a prescription for noncontrolled medications is not limited by federal law.

_____

_____ 10. Only authorized individuals are allowed to enter the prescription processing areas.

_____

_____ 11. On a prescription for a controlled substance, the lower the number of the drug schedule, the lower the potential for abuse of the drug.

_____

_____ 12. A professional is held accountable for his or her actions while on the job, must maintain an ethical standard of behavior, must clearly and concisely communicate with customers and other health care providers, and must be able to work as a team member and in a fast-paced environment.

_____

_____ 13. Ethics is the study of moral values or principles, and a professional is an individual qualified to perform the activities of a specific operation.

_____

_____ 14. All health care facilities had until April 14, 2003, to comply with the rules of national standards set in place by HIPAA.

_____

_____ 15. To keep up with the rising demand for pharmaceutical products and services, technicians will play a much greater role to support pharmaceutical care.

_____

_____ 16. Teamwork is also necessary for the smooth operation of the entire pharmacy.

_____

Multiple Choice

_____ 1. There are more than _____ community pharmacies across the United States.

A. 40,000   C. 60,000
B. 50,000   D. 70,000

_____ 2. Approximately _____ prescriptions are dispensed each year in the United States.

A. 2 billion   C. 6 billion
B. 4 billion   D. 8 billion

_____ 3. When a patient needs counseling, the only person who can legally do so is the:

    A. store manager.   C. pharmacist.

    B. pharmacy technician.   D. cashier.

_____ 4. Schedule III and IV can be refilled a maximum of:

    A. 1 refill in 6 months.   C. 5 refills in 6 months.

    B. 3 refills in 6 months.   D. 7 refills in 6 months.

_____ 5. Each pharmacy must have a refrigerator to store drugs that are required to be kept at temperatures between:

    A. 2 and 8 degrees.

    B. –6 and 0 degrees.

    C. 8 and 24 degrees.

    D. It does not matter, as long as the drug is kept on the top shelf.

_____ 6. Three areas in the pharmacy in which computerized systems can be used are:

    A. prescription dispensing and associated record maintenance.

    B. clinical support and accounting.

    C. business management.

    D. all the above.

_____ 7. A pharmacy technician needs to:

    A. be genuinely interested in helping people.   C. put the needs of others first.

    B. be warm and caring.   D. all the above.

Short Answer

1. List all the component parts that must be on a prescription.

_____

_____

_____

_____

_____

2. When is it acceptable to not use a child-resistant container when filling a prescription?

_____

_____

_____

_____

_____

3. Discuss the roles and responsibilities of pharmacy technicians.

_____

_____

_____

_____

_____

Advanced Pharmacy

Matching

Match the term with its definition.

_____ 1. automatic dispensing system

_____ 2. blended dose system

_____ 3. central fill pharmacy

_____ 4. drug distribution system

_____ 5. enteral nutrition

_____ 6. home health care pharmacy

_____ 7. hospice

_____ 8. Internet pharmacy

_____ 9. long-term care

_____ 10. long-term care pharmacy org

_____ 11. mail-order pharmacy

_____ 12. modular cassette

A. A drug distribution system that provides medication in its final unit of use form

B. A group of medications provided to a hospice patient by the hospice pharmacy to provide a "start" in treatment for most urgent problems that can develop during the last days or weeks of life

C. An intravenous feeding that supplies all the nutrients necessary for life

D. A safe and economical way of distributing a drug

E. A high-volume pharmacy that fills prescriptions for a number of individual pharmacies

F. A drug distribution system that combines a unit-of-use medication package with a non-unit-dose drug distribution system

G. A drug dispensing system that is computer or robot based

H. An established commercial website that enables a patient to obtain medications by way of the Internet

I. Originally a facility, usually within a hospital, intended to care for the terminally ill, in particular, by providing physical comfort to the patient and emotional support and counseling to the patient and the family; currently hospice care is also provided in home settings.

J. A licensed pharmacy that uses the mail or other carriers to deliver prescriptions to patients

K. An organization involving a licensed professional pharmacy or practice that provides medications and clinical services to long-term care facilities and their residents

L. A range of health and health-related support services provided over an extended period of time

_____ 13. modified unit dose system

_____ 14. multiple medication package

_____ 15. nuclear pharmacy

_____ 16. parenteral nutrition

_____ 17. radiopharmaceutical

_____ 18. reagent kit

_____ 19. specialty mail-order pharmacy

_____ 20. starter kit

_____ 21. total parenteral nutrition

_____ 22. unit-dose system

M. The practice of pharmacy that provides medications, home health care products and services, and pharmaceutical care to patients at home

N. Feedings given through a tube passed directly into the stomach or intestines

O. A mail-order pharmacy that concentrates on specific areas of the prescription drug market

P. Vials containing particular compounds, usually in freeze-dried form used in nuclear pharmacy

Q. A drug that is or has been made to be radioactive

R. A combination of amino acids, dextrose, fats, vitamins, minerals, electrolytes, and water administered intravenously

S. A pharmacy that is specially licensed to work with radioactive materials

T. A medication package in which all medications for a specific medication time are package together

U. A drug distribution system that combines unit-dose medications blister packaged onto a multiple dose card.

V. These cassettes contain either one-week or two-week medication strips that also contain reserve closes in a narrow plastic slidetray design.

True/False

_____ 1. Pharmacy technicians are trained to work in various care delivery areas, including inpatient care, homecare, ambulatory care, mail-order pharmacy, and more advanced areas, such as nuclear medicine and chemotherapy.

_____

_____ 2. There are now more acute care beds than long-term facility beds.

_____

_____ 3. Prolongation of life expectancy has created a totally new set of problems for the health care system.

_____

_____ 4. Pharmacy technicians should be familiar with the various types of drug distributions used in the long-term care pharmacy setting.

_____

_____ 5. Central fill pharmacy is a sterile compounding practice that is similar (but not identical) to a hospital pharmacy practice.

_____

_____ 6. There are two types of nutritional therapy provided by home infusion pharmacy: parenteral and enteral.

_____

_____ 7. A hospice pharmacy cannot be part of a traditional community pharmacy.

_____

_____ 8. The term *ambulatory care* includes a range of services such as outpatient pharmacies, emergency departments, primary care clinics, specialty clinics, ambulatory care centers, and family practice groups.

_____

_____ 9. Disadvantages of mail-order pharmacy include medication waste, lack of personal contact, increases in medication errors, and time delays.

_____

_____ 10. Disadvantages of central fill pharmacies include reduced costs, provision of patients with more options concerning their prescription, and allowance of local pharmacists at individual pharmacies to have more time for patient counseling.

_____

_____ 11. Legitimate Internet pharmacies operate with extremely rigid safeguards to ensure that their customers receive the best-quality pharmacy care and counseling.

_____

_____ 12. Iodine-131 is used to treat hyperthyroidism, as well as ovarian and prostate cancer.

_____

_____ 13. The pharmacist in a centralized nuclear pharmacy inherently spends considerable time preparing and dispensing radiopharmaceuticals.

_____

_____ 14. Because of advances in medical science and technology, people are living longer, resulting in the need for more long-term care than ever before.

_____

_____ 15. Hospice differs primarily from home health care in that the hospice patient is terminally ill.

_____

Multiple Choice

_____ 1. One of the fastest-growing parts of the health care market is:

A. home health care pharmacy.　　　　　　C. central fill pharmacy.
B. radioactive pharmacy.　　　　　　　　　D. Internet pharmacy.

_____ 2. The major sources of payment for home health care services are:

A. Medicare.　　　　　　　　　　　　　　　C. Tricare.
B. Medicaid.　　　　　　　　　　　　　　　D. both A and B.

_____ 3. TPNs consist of:

A. amino acid and dextrose.　　　　　　　　C. vitamins and trace elements.
B. fats and electrolytes.　　　　　　　　　　D. all the above.

_____ 4. Hospice pharmacy services can be divided into two areas:

A. management services and support services.　　C. inpatient and outpatient services.
B. clinical services and dispensing services.　　　D. none of the above.

_____ 5. Ambulatory care services provide:

A. mobile imaging.　　　　　　　　　　　　C. dialysis centers.
B. rehabilitation.　　　　　　　　　　　　　D. all the above.

Short Answer

1. List several types of home health care services that may be available.

_____

_____

_____

_____

_____

2. Give three examples of infusion therapies.

_____

_____

_____

_____

3. What are the three types of radiation that can be released by a radionuclide?

_____

_____

_____

_____

4. List the nine general areas involved in nuclear pharmacy practice.

_____

_____

_____

_____

Extemporaneous Prescription Compounding

Matching

Match the term to its definition.

_____ 1. compounding slab

_____ 2. conical graduates

_____ 3. counter balance

_____ 4. cylindrical graduates

_____ 5. electronic balance

_____ 6. elixir

_____ 7. emulsion

_____ 8. extemporaneous compounding

_____ 9. geometric dilution

_____ 10. levigate

_____ 11. meniscus

_____ 12. mortar

_____ 13. pestle

A. Meaning "moon-shaped body," indicates that the level of the liquid will be slightly higher at the edges

B. A solid device that is used to crush or grind material in a mortar

C. A liquid dosage form in which active ingredients are dissolved in a liquid vehicle

D. Solid, small, and usually cylindrically molded or compressed tablets

E. Devices used for measuring liquids that have wide tops and wide bases and taper from the top to the bottom

F. To grind into a smooth substance with moisture

G. A two-pan device that may be used for weighing small amounts of drugs (not more than 120 g)

H. The preparation, mixing, assembling, packaging, and labeling of a drug product based on a prescription order from a licensed practitioner for the individual patient

I. A plate made of ground glass with a hard, flat, and nonabsorbent surface for mixing compounds

J. To reduce a fine powder by friction

K. When mixing agents, the medicament is first mixed with an equal weight of diluent. A further quantity of diluent equal in weight to the mixture is then incorporated. This process is repeated until all the diluent has been mixed in.

L. A device capable of weighing much larger quantities, up to about 5 kg. It is a double-pan balance.

M. A cup-shaped vessel in which materials are ground or crushed

_____ 14. pipette

N. A suspension containing two different liquids and an agent that holds them together

_____ 15. solution

O. Devices used for measuring liquids that have narrow diameters that are the same from top to base

_____ 16. solvent

P. The weight of an empty capsule used to compare with the full capsule

_____ 17. suspension

Q. A liquid dosage form that contains solid drug particles floating in a liquid medium

_____ 18. tablet triturate

R. A long, thin, calibrated hollow tube, which is made of glass used for measuring liquids

_____ 19. tare

S. Sweetened liquid containing alcohol and water

_____ 20. triturate

T. The liquid substance in which another substance is being dissolved

True/False

Indicate whether the statement is true or false. If false, rewrite the statement to make it true.

_____ 1. An electronic balance and/or a Class A prescription balance is used when weighing amounts of 120 g or less.

_____

_____ 2. A counter balance is used for weighing larger quantities, but is not to be used for prescription compounding.

_____

_____ 3. Glass mortars and pestles are preferred when mixing liquids, while porcelain is best used when triturating crystals, granules, and powders.

_____

_____ 4. Spatulas made of rubber or plastic need not be cleaned between uses.

_____

_____ 5. Many state boards of pharmacy have a minimum list of equipment for prescription compounding.

_____

_____ 6. Emulsions, elixirs, creams, pastes, gels are a few examples of extemporaneous compounds.

_____

_____ 7. Sterile drugs must be prepared in clean room conditions.

_____

_____ 8. In the preparation of I.V. admixtures, quality control is essential, but documentation is not necessary.

_____

_____ 9. Creams are water-based, and ointments are oil-based.

_____

_____ 10. Two methods for the creation of emulsions are the "dry gum" and "wet gum" methods. They are also known as the Continental and English methods.

_____

Multiple Choice

_____ 1. In a community pharmacy the dosage form repackaged regularly is:

   A. liquids.   C. capsules.
   B. tablets.   D. all of the above.

_____ 2. _____ are prepared using the punch method.

   A. Capsules   C. Ointments
   B. Solutions   D. Tablets

_____ 3. _____ are the most frequently compounded form of medication.

   A. Creams   C. Tablets
   B. Gels   D. Liquids

_____ 4. Which of the following is not a semisolid dosage form?

   A. Pastes   C. Suppositories
   B. Creams   D. Ointments

_____ 5. Which of the following are used in nonsterile compounding?

   A. Mortars and pestles
   B. Slabs and spatulas
   C. Cylindrical and conical graduates
   D. Pipettes
   E. All of the above

Short Answer

1. What might the difference be in the compounding of nonsterile products in a hospital pharmacy versus a local community pharmacy?

_____

_____

_____

_____

_____

2. Are there any additional skills or training necessary to be able to compound sterile and nonsterile preparations? If so, describe.

_____

_____

_____

_____

_____

3. Who is responsible in the preparation of compounds, the technician, the pharmacist, or both?

_____

_____

_____

_____

_____

4. Why are proper documentation and quality control important in compounding?

_____

_____

_____

_____

_____

5. What are some differences between sterile and nonsterile compounding, and why?

_____

_____

_____

_____

_____

CHAPTER 22

Sterile Compounding

Matching

Match the term with its definition.

_____ 1. aseptic technique

_____ 2. autoclave

_____ 3. beyond use date

_____ 4. chemical sterilization

_____ 5. conjunctiva

_____ 6. dry heat sterilization

_____ 7. gas sterilization

_____ 8. laminar airflow hood

_____ 9. medical asepsis

_____ 10. parenteral

_____ 11. sanitization

_____ 12. sterilization

_____ 13. surgical asepsis

_____ 14. total parenteral nutrition

A. Mucous membranes of the eyes

B. A method of cleaning equipment used for instruments that cannot be exposed to the high temperatures of steam sterilization

C. Date after which a product is no longer effective and should not be used

D. A sterilizing machine. It uses a combination of heat, steam, and pressure to sterilize equipment.

E. Preparing and handling sterile products in a manner that prevents microbial contamination

F. A method of sterilization that uses heated dry air at a temperature of 320 degrees to 365 degrees for 90 minutes to 3 hours

G. The use of a gas such as ethylene oxide to sterilize medical equipment

H. A system of circulating filtered air in parallel-flowing planes in hospitals or other health care facilities. The system reduces the risk of airborne contamination and exposure to chemical pollutants in surgical theaters, food preparation areas, hospital pharmacies, and laboratories.

I. Nutrition system involving the intravenous infusion directly into a vein of lipids, proteins, electrolytes, sugars, salts, vitamins, and essential elements

J. The complete destruction of organisms before they enter the body

K. Complete destruction of all forms of microbial life

L. A process of cleaning to remove undesirable debris

M. Complete destruction of organisms after they leave the body

N. Bypassing the skin and gastrointestinal tract; injected

True/False

Indicate if the statement is true or false. If false, rewrite the statement to make it true.

_____ 1. Parenteral products are injected directly into body tissue through the skin and vein.

_____

_____ 2. Sterile preparations must be kept pure and free from biological, chemical, and physical contaminants.

_____

_____ 3. It is not necessary for parenteral products to be isotonic.

_____

_____ 4. It is not necessary for parenteral products to be chemically, physically, or microbiologically stable.

_____

_____ 5. The single most important means of preventing the spread of infection is frequent and effective hand hygiene by all health care workers.

_____

_____ 6. Hibiclens is an example of a good antimicrobial soap containing chlorhexidine.

_____

_____ 7. Proper hand washing depends on two factors: water temperature and chlorine levels in the water used.

_____

_____ 8. The use of disposable instruments when working with human blood or giving injections minimizes the need for sanitization, disinfection, and sterilization.

_____

_____ 9. Living tissue surfaces such as skin can be sterilized.

_____

_____ 10. Surgical asepsis requires sterile hand washing, sterile gloves, special handling procedures, and sterilization of materials.

_____

_____ 11. Gas sterilization is not commonly used in hospitals that have room-sized gas sterilization chambers.

_____

_____ 12. Catheters are inserted into veins for direct vascular system access.

_____

_____ 13. Sharps containers are a rigid plastic containers used for sharps such as needles and scalpel blades.

_____

_____ 14. 70% isopropyl alcohol is used for cleaning surfaces.

_____

_____ 15. The controlled area should be a limited-access area sufficiently separated from other pharmacy operations to minimize the potential for contamination that could result from the unnecessary flow of materials and personnel into and out of the area.

_____

_____ 16. The air moves at a rate to 60 to 75 linear feet per minute, with very little turbulence, at a uniform velocity.

_____

_____ 17. HEPA stands for "high efficiency particulate air filter."

_____

_____ 18. HEPA filters cannot be cleaned or recycled and must be replaced every 3 to 5 years on average.

_____

_____ 19. In the pharmacy, it is important that the pharmacist ensures the stability, compatibility, and safety of the mixture.

_____

_____ 20. The most common sterile irrigations include gentamicin irrigation solution and surgical antibiotic solution.

_____

_____ 21. The process for compounding ophthalmics properly takes from 3 to 5 weeks.

_____

Multiple Choice

_____ 1. Parenteral products must have the following unique qualities:

   A. must be sterile   C. free from visible particles
   B. be free from contamination by endotoxins   D. all the above

_____ 2. A disadvantage of parenteral administration is that:

   A. it's painless.   C. there's no risk of tissue toxicity from local irritation.

   B. asepsis is required at administration.   D. all the above

_____ 3. Important properties of parenteral preparations that must be considered include:

   A. compatibility.   C. both A and B.
   B. osmolality.   D. none of the above.

_____ 4. Methods of sterilization include:

   A. application of steam under pressure.   C. chemicals and radiation.
   B. dry heat and gas.   D. all the above.

_____ 5. Used to remove particulates and microorganisms from solutions:

   A. filters   C. filter straws
   B. filter needles   D. none of the above

_____ 6. Laminar airflow hoods are used to prepare sterile compounds by circulating air through HEPA filters to remove _____ of possible contaminants.

   A. 50%   C. 99%
   B. 70%   D. None of the above

_____ 7. Sneezing produces _____ aerosol droplets.

   A. 100,000   C. 300,000
   B. 200,000   D. 400,000

Short Answer

1. List the six categories injections are classified in for administration purposes.

_____

_____

_____

_____

_____

2. Discuss the two types of asepsis.

_____

_____

_____

_____

3. List several pieces of equipment used in sterile compounding.

_____

_____

_____

_____

_____

4. What are the two types of laminar airflow hoods?

_____

_____

_____

_____

5. What is pharmacokinetics?

_____

_____

_____

_____

_____

6. What is the difference between solubility and compatibility?

_____

_____

_____

_____

_____

Administrative

CHAPTER 23

Management of Pharmacy Operations

Matching

Match the term with its definition.

_____ 1. bar code

_____ 2. batch repackaging

_____ 3. cost analysis

_____ 4. cost-benefit analysis

_____ 5. cost control

_____ 6. group purchasing

_____ 7. independent purchasing

_____ 8. inventory

_____ 9. invoice

_____ 10. prime supplier

_____ 11. time purchase

_____ 12. unit-of-use packaging

_____ 13. want book

A. A list of drugs and devices that routinely need to be reordered

B. A form describing a purchase and the amount due

C. The stock of medications a pharmacy keeps immediately on hand

D. The director of pharmacy or buyer directly contacts and negotiates pricing with pharmaceutical manufactures

E. Many hospitals working together to negotiate with pharmaceutical manufacturers to get better prices and benefits based upon the ability to promise high committed volumes

F. The implementation of managerial efforts to achieve cost objectives

G. The procedure of evaluating cost and benefits of only those programs whose benefits are found to supersede the costs

H. All information regarding the disbursements of an activity, department, program, or agency

I. The reassembling of a specific dosage and dosage form of medication at a given time

J. Placing a code on packaging to help standardize and regulate inventory control

K. The packaging from bulk containers into patient-specific containers

L. Establishment of a relationship with a single supplier to obtain lower prices

M. The time that the purchase order was made

True/False

_____ 1. Pharmacy practice has remained unchanged for the last several years.

_____ 2. The need for pharmacy managers has decreased.

_____ 3. An integral part of the cost control process is the establishment of priorities for the implementation of cost control programs.

_____ 4. Decisions of cost control should be based on the total cost of a system such as supplies, personnel, overhead, and others.

_____ 5. Overhead, central pharmacy administration, and fringe benefits are examples of indirect costs.

_____ 6. Indirect costs do not relate to morbidity and mortality.

_____ 7. The larger the purchase, the lower the prices.

_____ 8. Regular drugs, devices, and supplies may be ordered electronically by fax or telephone or online by computer.

_____ 9. Colored or dated price stickers are another high-tech and effective manual technique used for ordering.

_____ 10. After products are received and checked, they must be placed in an appropriate storage location.

_____ 11. The FDA has helped to direct the implementation of bar coding so that patient safety is kept in mind.

_____ 12. For damaged or incorrect shipments or expired medications, the manufacturer should be notified immediately and a returned merchandise authorization should be requested for the return of the rejected shipment.

_____ 13. Under the federal Food, Drug, and Cosmetic Act, the FDA can request a recall if a drug manufacturer is not willing to remove dangerous drugs from the market without the FDA's written request.

_____ 14. Files must be kept on hard copy; computer disks are not permitted.

_____ 15. All records for wholesale distributors need to be kept separate and distinct from the records for the rest of the pharmacy operation.

_____ 16. The amount of medication that is repackaged into the patient container is generally predicated on the course of therapy.

_____

_____ 17. Pharmacies survive by providing products and services that their customers need.

_____

_____ 18. Cost control is central to the pharmacy's success.

_____

_____ 19. Expired, deteriorated, or contaminated drugs in all pharmacy areas should be considered "nonreusable" and should be removed immediately from usable stock either by direct disposal into the sink, trash, toilet, or biohazard bags or by return to the pharmacy stockroom for credit.

_____

_____ 20. Expired compounded or repackaged pharmaceuticals can be returned and recycled.

_____

_____ 21. The "want book" is based on the average sales ratio.

_____

Multiple Choice

_____ 1. Managers are responsible for:

A. planning.   C. controlling resources.
B. organizing.   D. all of the above.

_____ 2. The ultimate goal of an effective health program is to offer the best quality services for the most:

A. number of people.   C. customer satisfaction.
B. affordable prices.   D. sales.

_____ 3. Direct costs include:

A. prevention.   C. treatment.
B. rehabilitation.   D. all the above.

_____ 4. One of the most important parts of the pharmacy operation is:

A. receiving.   C. lunchtime.
B. spending.   D. none of the above.

_____ 5. One of the simplest and most widely used methods of inventory control is:

A. the want book.   C. prime supplier.
B. group purchasing.   D. independent purchasing.

Short Answer

1. What are the purposes for a cost-analysis study?

_____

_____

_____

_____

_____

2. What are three factors that affect costs in a hospital industry or community pharmacy?

_____

_____

_____

_____

_____

3. List three disadvantages of using a prime supplier.

_____

_____

_____

_____

_____

4. What are the four basic functions of drug packages?

_____

_____

_____

_____

_____

Health Insurance

Matching

Match the term with its definition.

_____ 1. beneficiary

_____ 2. CHAMPVA

_____ 3. coinsurance

_____ 4. contract

_____ 5. co-payment

_____ 6. deductible

_____ 7. dependents

_____ 8. eligibility

_____ 9. health insurance

_____ 10. Medicaid

A. The individual or organization protected in case of loss under the terms of an insurance policy. The subscriber is known as an insured or a member, policyholder, or recipient.

B. The premium is the cost of the coverage that the insurance policy contains and may vary greatly depending on the age and health of the individual and the type of insurance protection.

C. Prior authorization; many private insurance companies and prepaid health plans have certain requirements that must be met before they will approve diagnostic testing, hospital admissions, inpatient or outpatient surgical procedure; specific procedures, and specific treatment or medications.

D. Some patients or individuals have exclusion health insurance policies. Some types of exclusions are AIDS, attempted suicide, cancer, losses due to injury on the job, and pregnancy.

E. Payment by the insurer or by the patient of more than the amount due

F. A government-funded program that pays for health coverage for people over age 65, and certain other persons

G. An organization or corporation that pays medical claims for patients; it reimburses providers directly, with patients making only required copayments.

H. The amount of time from the date of service to the date a claim can be filed with the insurance company

I. Elimination period; the period of time that an individual must wait to become eligible for insurance coverage before coverage commences or for a specific benefit

J. A health care program serving active duty service members, members of the National Guard, retirees, their families, survivors, and selected former spouses worldwide

_____ 11. Medicare

_____ 12. overpayment

_____ 13. policy limitation

_____ 14. preauthorization

_____ 15. premium

_____ 16. subscriber

_____ 17. third-party payer

_____ 18. time limit

_____ 19. TRICARE

_____ 20. waiting period

K. An insurance policy; this is a legally enforceable agreement.

L. An arrangement in which the insured must pay either a fixed amount or a percentage of the cost of medical services covered by the insurer

M. A comprehensive health care program in which the Office of Veterans' Affairs shares the cost of covered health care services and supplies with eligible beneficiaries

N. A person designated by an insurance policy to receive benefits or funds

O. The spouse and children of the insured who are also covered under the terms of the policy

P. A specific amount of money that must be paid yearly before the policy benefits begin

Q. The responsibility of the insured to make a payment of a specified amount at the time of treatment or purchase of a prescription

R. The determination of the exact coverage the insured is entitled to

S. A contract purchased by individuals or employers that agrees to pay the costs of specified medical and related expenses

T. A government-funded health cost assistance program that pays for health services and pharmacy expenses for enrolled U.S. citizens who cannot afford to pay for their own health care.

True/False

Indicate whether the statement is true or false. If false, rewrite the statement to make it true.

_____ 1. Medicaid covers those who are blind, disabled, orphaned, or underaged parents.

_____

_____ 2. The higher the deductible is, the higher the cost of the policy, and the lower the deductible, the lower the cost of the policy.

_____

_____ 3. In group insurance, the employer is known as the insured, and the employees are the risks.

_____

_____ 4. The purpose of health insurance is to help offset some of the high costs accrued from an injury or illness.

_____

_____ 5. Pharmacy technicians do not need to be familiar with different types of patient insurance coverage.

_____

_____ 6. Blue Cross and Blue Shield is a private insurer and not government run.

_____

_____ 7. HMOs were the first type of managed care organizations developed to control the expenditure of health care dollars and to manage patient care.

_____ 8. There are no time limitations set forth for the prompt reporting of workers' compensation cases.

_____ 9. An independent practice association is a closed-panel HMO.

_____ 10. Medicare is the smallest single medical benefits program in the United States.

_____ 11. Medicare Part B coverage is optional.

_____ 12. Medicaid premiums are paid for by Medicare Part B.

_____ 13. Medicare Part D is offered to all Medicare recipients to cover the costs of their medications.

_____ 14. When you first become eligible for Medicare, you may choose to join or not join Part E.

_____ 15. TRICARE requires that prescriptions be filled with generic products if they are available.

_____ 16. Paper claims involve use of the "universal claim" form known as CMS-1500.

_____ 17. Anyone who finds that his or her privacy has been compromised in any manner can file a complaint with the Department of Health and Human Services.

_____ 18. To prove fraud, two types of international actions must be proven: intent to practice the fraudulent act and intent to commit a major offense.

_____ 19. Most of the accounts receivable amounts are paid within 90 days after the date of service.

_____ 20. An important role of the pharmacy technician handling insurance billing is to follow up balances that are still outstanding and make sure that the responsible payer sends payment.

Multiple Choice

_____ 1. _____ is an agreement between a policyholder and a health plan.

A. Personal insurance
B. Medical insurance

C. Health and healing insurance
D. None of the above

_____ 2. The majority of patients, almost _____, have coverage from some type of insurance policy or other third-party payer.

    A. 64%   C. 84%

    B. 74%   D. 94%

_____ 3. Third-party insurances include:

    A. Blue Cross.   C. Medicaid.

    B. Medicare.   D. All the above.

_____ 4. A response and/or payment from Blue Cross Blue Shield may take up to _____ days.

    A. 45   C. 60

    B. 55   D. 90

_____ 5. During the past _____ decades, there have been many reforms of the health care system.

    A. five   C. seven

    B. six   D. eight

Short Answer

1. What is the Kaiser Foundation Health Plan?

_____

_____

_____

_____

_____

2. Give three examples of classes of drugs for which many insurance plans require preauthorization before accepting.

_____

_____

_____

_____

_____

3. What are the three options individuals have to consider under the TRICARE program?

_____

_____

_____

_____

_____

4. What are the HIPAA standard claims status category codes?

_____

_____

_____

_____

_____

5. What is an example of fraud?

_____

_____

_____

_____

_____

Documentation, Billing, and Collection

Matching

Match the term with its definition.

_____ 1. biennial inventories

_____ 2. collections

_____ 3. collections letter

_____ 4. dispersal records

_____ 5. Drug Enforcement Administration

_____ 6. invoice

_____ 7. legibility

_____ 8. medication reconciliation

_____ 9. National Council for Prescription Drug Programs

_____ 10. professional pharmacy services

_____ 11. protected health information

_____ 12. statement

_____ 13. electronic data interchange

A. The process of comparing a patient's medication orders to all of the medications that the patient has been taking

B. A request for payment, often covering several invoices during a specific time period

C. The degree to which something is able to be read based on its appearance

D. Complete lists of all products stored in a pharmacy, conducted every two years

E. Any information about a patient's health status, provision of health care, or payment for health care

F. All of the activities that a licensed pharmacy provides

G. A nonprofit organization representing every sector of the pharmacy industry; it develops standards and provides education about pharmacy-related topics.

H. A form that describes a purchase and the amount that is due

I. The structured transmission of data using electronic devices

J. A federal law enforcement agency that combats illegal drug use and smuggling both within the United States and abroad

K. Lists of all drugs dispensed from a pharmacy or removed for any reason

L. A document that notifies a customer that their bill is past due

M. All of the activities of handling patient accounting and following up to ensure timely payments

True/False

Indicate whether the statement is true or false. If false, rewrite the statement to make it true.

_____ 1. In pharmacy, documentation is not very important.

_____ 2. Electronic documentation can easily improve pharmacy service.

_____ 3. Electronic billing is not used in pharmacy due to the length of time it takes to enter patient information.

_____ 4. Medicare representatives can enter a hospital or a pharmacy to perform audits without warning, appointments, or search warrants.

_____ 5. If HIPAA confidentiality rules are broken, it can lead to termination of the pharmacy technician.

_____ 6. The mission of the NCPDP has been to create and promote voluntary standards for information transfer in prescription drug benefit program administration.

_____ 7. Federal law requires all personnel, including pharmacy technicians, to help manage controlled substances located in the workplace, but state law does not.

_____ 8. Ensuring confidentiality requirements while at the same time minimizing retrieval speed is important.

_____ 9. The majority of customers who come to a retail pharmacy for medications, devices, or other supplies have insurance that partially or completely covers them.

_____ 10. Hospital and retail pharmacies are a lot alike.

_____ 11. MAR stands for "medication administration record."

_____ 12. The staff of the hospital pharmacy have a lot of interaction with patients concerning billing and collections.

_____ 13. Pharmacies must clearly explain every patient's responsibilities for payments.

_____ 14. FACTA stands for Fair and Accurate Credit Transaction Act.

_____ 15. Pharmacy technicians are not responsible for documenting billing and reimbursement activities correctly in case of future audits.

Multiple Choice

_____ 1. Pharmacy technicians may be required to assist with many administrative tasks such as:

A. billing.

B. documentation.

C. reimbursements to patients.

D. all the above.

_____ 2. Under HIPAA regulation, pharmacy technicians are required to maintain patient:

A. costs.

B. confidentiality.

C. care.

D. all the above.

_____ 3. Controlled substances records must be kept a minimum of _____ years and some states require as long as _____ years.

A. 2 and 5.

B. 2 and 6.

C. 3 and 5.

D. 3 and 4.

_____ 4. DEA Form 222 is used to _____ controlled substances.

A. destroy

B. order and return

C. replace

D. report theft of

Short Answer

1. What are some reasons that would cause Medicare to audit a pharmacy or hospital?

_____

_____

_____

_____

_____

2. What are the six PCCF fields of information?

_____

_____

_____

_____

_____

3. What are the two most important acts that relate to collections?

_____

_____

_____

_____

_____

CHAPTER 26

Inventory Control

Matching

Match the term with its definition.

_____ 1. inventory

_____ 2. inventory control

_____ 3. inventory turnover rate

_____ 4. perpetual inventory system

_____ 5. point-of-sale master

_____ 6. receiving report

_____ 7. want book

A. Inventory control systems that allow monthly drug use reviews

B. A list of drugs and devices that routinely need to be reordered

C. The stock of medications a pharmacy keeps immediately on hand

D. A document showing received items; it should match the purchase order exactly.

E. An inventory control system that allows inventory to be tracked as it is used

F. A mathematical calculation of the number of times the average inventory is replaced over a period of time (usually annually)

G. Controlling the amount of product on hand to maximize the return on investment

True/False

Indicate whether the statement is true or false. If false, rewrite the statement to make it true.

_____ 1. Improper inventory control systems help to streamline the hectic activities of the pharmacies of today.

_____

_____ 2. Point-of-sale masters aid in inventory control by accurately controlling pharmacy stock and increasing the amount of customers and transactions that can be handled, enhancing the pharmacy's operational abilities.

_____

_____ 3. Inventory control is of vital importance because a pharmacy must have the correct inventory to properly serve its patients.

_____

_____ 4. The two goals of effective inventory control are minimizing total inventory investment and carrying the right mix of products to satisfy patient demand.

_____ 5. Inventory turnover rate equals purchases over a period of time multiplied by the average inventory for the period.

_____ 6. The lead time is assumed to be "one," as orders to replenish stock are made when the inventory level reduces to one. This number is set and never changes.

_____ 7. The medication master file contains all of the information needed for ordering, inventory, pricing, and distribution of pharmaceuticals.

_____ 8. The minimum/maximum-level system involves ordering products when a specified minimum level is reached, not to exceed a maximum amount of storable products—this means the total amount that the pharmacy can actually have on hand.

_____ 9. Miscalculating finances can lead to the perception that the pharmacy is being managed incorrectly or even illegally.

_____ 10. The state board of pharmacy has no power to start an investigation if financial statements seem incorrect or possibly suspect.

_____ 11. When opening a received package, pharmacy staff members must be extremely accurate in verifying the items received.

_____ 12. Other methods of stocking involve using alphabetic organization by using each drug's generic name or, less commonly, its trade name.

_____ 13. Drug formularies are lists or catalogs of drugs that are approved for use either within a hospital or for reimbursement by a third-party payer.

_____ 14. Automated dispensing systems are becoming obsolete in the dispensing of drugs in a pharmacy.

_____ 15. Most automated dispensing systems do not comply with HIPAA regulations.

_____ 16. Efficient management of expired stock should be a regular part of pharmacy practice, and may easily be accomplished by the use of computerized inventory control.

_____ 17. Purchase orders authorize items to be purchased from vendors, and include the price of each item.

_____ 18. Automation in the pharmacy is far from the wave of the future in pharmacy. It is very unrealistic.

_____ 19. Formularies are revised every year, and a process must be in place for these revisions.

_____

_____ 20. The restrictive use of formularies has led to a number of important ethical questions.

_____

Multiple Choice

_____ 1. Several important factors and issues with regard to inventory are:

A. How much inventory should be maintained?   C. Where should inventory be stored?
B. When should inventory levels be adjusted?   D. All the above

_____ 2. A common inventory management error made is:

A. miscounting the final inventory.   C. correct storage.
B. creating labels that are not easily read.   D. both A and B.

_____ 3. One of the simplest and most widely used methods of inventory control is:

A. the want book.   C. perpetual inventory system.
B. point of sale.   D. computerized inventory system.

_____ 4. Board regulation requires that a pharmacist should keep a _____ of each controlled substance in Schedule II, which has been received, dispensed, or disposed of.

A. point-of-sale master   C. want inventory
B. perpetual inventory   D. None of the above

_____ 5. An advantage of computerized inventory control systems is:

A. time saving for the pharmacy and the business office.
B. saving money for insurance companies.
C. better tracking for management statistics.
D. all the above.

Short Answer

1. Discuss common management systems listed in this chapter.

_____

_____

_____

_____

_____

2. What is the information that must be specified when ordering inventory?

_____

_____

_____

_____

_____

3. What do you think is the most effective inventory system? Which one would you use in your pharmacy?

_____

_____

_____

_____

_____

CHAPTER 27

Computers in the Pharmacy

Matching

Match the term with its definition.

_____ 1. automated touch-tone response system

_____ 2. central processing unit

_____ 3. data

_____ 4. file

_____ 5. hardware

_____ 6. input devices

_____ 7. memory

_____ 8. modem

_____ 9. output devices

_____ 10. personal digital assistant

_____ 11. software

_____ 12. touch screen

_____ 13. users

_____ 14. computer

A. The individuals who work with computers regularly

B. A monitor with a touch-sensitive surface, in which the touch of a finger makes a selection as a mouse pointer does

C. A set of electronic instructions that tell the computer what to do

D. A device used to transfer information from one computer to another

E. A piece of programmable equipment that stores, retrieves, and processes data

F. A system in which the patient can call in an order or refill a prescription and the system routes the fill orders to the proper pharmacy and assigns each order a place in the order-fulfillment sequence

G. The parts of the computer that you can touch

H. A set of data or a program that has been given a name

I. A handheld device that runs on its own battery power so that it may be used anywhere

J. The ability of the computer to store and retrieve data

K. Any piece of equipment that allows data to exit the computer system

L. Any piece of equipment that allows data to be entered into the computer system

M. The raw facts the computer can manipulate

N. The part of the computer that does the computations

True/False

Indicate whether the statement is true or false. If false, rewrite the statement to make it true.

_____ 1. Computers have revolutionized the pharmacy world and are the main component of pharmacy practice.

_____ 2. Computers increase the cost of any operation that involves the processing of information.

_____ 3. The overall goal in the use of better computer applications in the pharmacy is to reduce errors.

_____ 4. The CPU is the "liver" of the computers.

_____ 5. Electronic medical record systems provide better control over distinct patient identification, correct information, and identifying codes to help locate a specific record among large numbers of other patient records.

_____ 6. The most common device used to input information into the computer is the keyboard.

_____ 7. The monitor is the most-used output device on a computer.

_____ 8. Displays use tiny dots of light called "panels" to make up the various graphical components on their screens.

_____ 9. Flat panel touch screen monitors take up less counter space than full-sized monitors, and installation takes only two days to complete.

_____ 10. A scanner is a device that can convert printed matter and images to information that can be interpreted by the computer.

_____ 11. The word *modem* is a blend of two words: *modulator* and *demodulator*.

_____ 12. Inkjet printers are preferred over laser printers and other types of printers because of their speed, precision, and economy.

_____ 13. Computer software can be classified into operation systems and applications.

_____ 14. Examples of drug information software commonly used in the pharmacy include Micromedex and Lexicomp.

_____ 15. OBRA stands for Omnibus Budget Reconciliation Act.

_____ 16. The National Mail Order Pharmacy assists millions of active-duty service members and their families, as well as military retirees.

_____

_____ 17. Hospitals have highly sophisticated diagnostic capabilities, but providers often do not have access to the results.

_____

_____ 18. PDAs are usually the size of a bowling ball.

_____

_____ 19. New technology, governmental policies, and consumer demands all create the need for improved information systems.

_____

_____ 20. Pharmacists should provide regular training updates and appropriate resources for all current and future staff members.

_____

_____ 21. The future of the pharmacy profession is assured with the use of computerization, which is integral to both the pharmacy management and patient satisfaction that can be provided.

_____

Multiple Choice

_____ 1. Computers gather and analyze data from which:

A. tables can be made.
B. graphics can be made.
C. models and designs can be made.
D. all the above.

_____ 2. RAM stands for:

A. ready access memory.
B. random access memory.
C. reasonable access memory.
D. reliable access memory.

_____ 3. _____ allow many different computer components and devices to be interconnected.

A. USB connectors
B. Keyboards
C. Hardware
D. Touch screens

_____ 4. Input devices include:

A. keyboards and mouse.
B. touch screens and scanners.
C. modems.
D. all the above.

_____ 5. Popular automated distribution systems include:

A. Archimedes and Diagnosaurus.
B. Lasertec and Pillwatch.
C. Pyxis and Omnicell.
D. HIPAA and Jointcontrol.

Short Answer

1. What are the benefits of an optical mouse?

_____

_____

_____

_____

_____

2. What are the most often accessed topics via touch screen programs?

_____

_____

_____

_____

_____

3. What are two questions to consider when a physician order-entry system is implemented?

_____

_____

_____

_____

_____

4. List five details that must be protected in reference to patients' privacy.

_____

_____

_____

_____

_____

Communications

Matching

Match the term with its definition.

_____ 1. compensation

_____ 2. apathy

_____ 3. autonomy

_____ 4. channels

_____ 5. consumer

_____ 6. communication

_____ 7. decode

_____ 8. defense mechanism

_____ 9. denial

_____ 10. displacement

_____ 11. expressive aphasia

_____ 12. external noise

_____ 13. internal noise

A. A physical limitation after certain neurological injuries, which leaves the person incapable of understanding all that is said

B. A defense mechanism of keeping out and ejecting or banishing from consciousness an unacceptable idea or impulse

C. A psychological defense mechanism in which confrontation with a personal problem or with reality is avoided by denying the existence of the problem or reality

D. Behavior based on body of knowledge and ethical standards to serve the public

E. A psychoanalytic defense mechanism through which irrational behavior, motives, or feelings are made to appear reasonable

F. The sharing of information, ideas, thoughts, and feelings

G. A lack of feeling, emotion, interest, or concern

H. An individual's beliefs or prejudices that interfere with decoding a message

I. An unconscious defense mechanism in which unacceptable instinctual drives and wishes are modified into more personally and socially acceptable channels

J. Inability of an individual to form language and express his or her thoughts accurately even though thought processes are intact

K. An unconscious defense mechanism involving a return to earlier patterns of adaptation

L. A defense mechanism by which a repressed complex in the individual is denied and conceived as belonging to another person, such as when faults that the person tends to commit are perceived in or attributed to others

M. Spoken words, written messages, and body language

_____ 14. prejudice

_____ 15. professionalism

_____ 16. projection

_____ 17. rationalism

_____ 18. receptive aphasia

_____ 19. regression

_____ 20. repression

_____ 21. sarcasm

_____ 22. sexual harassment

_____ 23. sublimation

N. Translation of a message by the receiver into what is perceived to be said

O. Intentional, clearly understood statements or intentional, clearly understood action that causes another to feel that his or her job is at risk if the sexual advances are rejected

P. The person coming to you for the filling of prescriptions or the purchase of over-the-counter remedies for a wide variety of situations

Q. Hostile and cruel language intended to hurt someone

R. An unconscious mechanism by which an individual tries to make up for fancied or real deficiencies

S. A performed and unsubstantiated judgment or opinion about an individual or a group, either favorable or unfavorable

T. Tools an individual uses when required to deal with uncomfortable or threatening situations

U. The transfer of impulses from one expression to another, such as from fighting to talking

V. The right of an individual to make informed decisions for his or her own good

W. Physical noise such as typing or traffic that interferes with hearing a message

Match the term with its meaning.

_____ 1. sender

_____ 2. message

_____ 3. channel

_____ 4. receiver

_____ 5. feedback

A. The path that a message takes from the sender to the receiver

B. Verbal expressions, body language

C. The person who delivers a message through a variety of different channels

D. The person who decodes the message

E. Contains all necessary information

True/False

Indicate whether the statement is true or false. If false, rewrite the statement to make it true.

_____ 1. Feedback can be verbal expression or body language.

_____ 2. Feedback is sometimes called criticism.

_____ 3. Two kinds of noise are external noise and rational noise.

_____ 4. Proper diction and enunciation are not required for speaking clearly and accurately.

_____ 5. Verbal communication consists of just words.

_____

_____ 6. Pharmacy technicians need not have the ability to communicate effectively with supervisors, peers, or other heath care workers.

_____

_____ 7. Body language is an important part of nonverbal communication.

_____

_____ 8. Eye contact, hand gestures, and appearance are an integral part of nonverbal communication.

_____

_____ 9. As a technician, your only customers are ones with prescriptions.

_____

_____ 10. Technicians need to be familiar with the use of the telephone, fax machine, computers, and their programs.

_____

Fill in the Blank

1. The goal of all communication is _____.

2. Verbal communication also consists of _____, _____, and level of pitch, which determine the meaning of the message.

3. Excellent _____ communication skills are important in the pharmacy setting.

4. Most of our communicative transmissions are _____.

5. During a communication, posture can be described as _____ or _____.

Multiple Choice

_____ 1. Which of the following is not conducive to a good message?

    A. Clarity   C. Criticism
    B. Cohesiveness   D. Courtesy

_____ 2. Which of the following is not a guideline for giving feedback?

    A. Be specific   C. Be clear
    B. Be descriptive   D. Be disrespectful

_____ 3. Which of the following will a pharmacy technician use most often?

    A. Telecommunication conferences   C. One on one, face to face
    B. Voice and e-mail   D. Computers

_____ 4. Which of the following is the most important nonverbal communication skill?

    A. Hand gestures   C. Tone of voice
    B. Body language   D. Maintaining good eye contact

_____ 5. When taking pertinent information during a phone call from a doctor's office it is important to get at a minimum:

    A. name, address, phone number, and gender.   C. name, address, age, and phone number.
    B. name, date and time, and phone number.   D. name, sex, date and time, and address.

_____ 6. Sexual harassment can be:

A. physical or verbal.   C. gestures or images.

B. written or spoken.   D. all of the above.

A Personal Point of View

Speaking from my own personal experience, I can say that your tone of voice is very important, along with your choice of words. Eye contact makes the person you are talking to feel that they are the most important priority to you.

In my specialty, oncology, you learn that a touch, a look, your tone of voice can make all the difference in the world to your patient. That same philosophy of caring should be applied to every patient or customer that the pharmacy technician comes into contact with. It might seem or sound to you that this is not possible, but *it is*. If you truly love your chosen profession, with time your skills will become honed, and these skills will become automatic. You will be able to accomplish this task readily and easily.

Chapter 1: History of Pharmacy
Matching

Match the term to the definition.

1. B   2. C   3. A   4. D

Match the legislation with its description

1. C   2. E   3. D   4. A   5. G   6. F   7. B

True/False

1. T

2. T

3. F, The "Father of medicine" was *Hippocrates*.

4. T

5. T

6. F, William Proctor introduced *"control"* into the practice of pharmacy in America.

7. F, *Benjamin Franklin* started the fist hospital in America.

8. T

9. T

10. F, The field of pharmacy has been around *since the dawn of mankind*.

11. F, Dosage form refers to *the make up of a particular drug*.

12. T

13. T

14. T

15. T

Short Answer

1. formularies, dosage forms, pharmacy shops

2. leaves, mud, cool water, clay

3. It has evolved from simply preparing and dispensing medications to acting as a patient advocate.

4. centralized manufacture of pharmaceuticals, industrialized manufacturing of pharmaceuticals, retail pharmacies

Chapter 2: The Foundation of Pharmaceutical Care
Matching

Match the term with the definition.

1. A   2. D   3. B   4. C   5. E

Match the abbreviation with its full title.

1. D   2. F   3. A   4. E   5. G   6. B   7. C

True/False

1. T

2. F, The profession of pharmacy focuses on ensuring that patients *receive the proper medication for their specific medical conditions*.

3. T

4. F, Pharmacist education *requires two years of undergraduate study followed by four years of graduate study*.

5. T

6. T

7. F, Once a pharmacy technician obtains proper licensing, *continuing education is required as well as recertification*.

8. F, A *pharmacist* may council patients.

9. T

10. T

11. T

12. T

Short Answer

1. See Table 2-1

2. interpretation of the prescription; use of patient profiles; dispensing, labeling, storing, and delivering medications; drug calculations

3. Assisting the Pharmacist in Serving Patients, Maintaining Medication Inventory Control Systems, and Participating in the Administration and Management of the Pharmacy

139

4. a method used to eliminate or reduce the potential harm of the drug distributed; it optimizes safety for the patients

5. See pages 28 through 30

Multiple Choice

1. b   2. c   3. c   4. a   5. b   6. d   7. a   8. a

Chapter 3: Pharmacy Law and Ethics for Technicians
Matching

Match the term with the definition.

1. C   2. B   3. E   4. A   5. D   6. G
7. H   8. F   9. J   10. I   11. K

Match the legislation with its description.

1. C   2. D   3. F   4. B   5. A   6. H
7. G   8. E   9. I   10. J

True/False

1. T

2. F, Judicial law results from *court decisions*, whereas statute results from action by the *legislature*.

3. T

4. T

5. F, The FDA oversees all domestic and imported food, bottled water, and wine beverages with less than **7%** alcohol.

6. T

7. T

8. F, A National Drug Code (NDC) identifies *the manufacturer or distributor, the drug formulation, and the size and type of its packaging*.

9. F, OSHA stands for Occupational Safety and Health Act

10. T

11. T

12. T

13. F, The DEA *must be* notified is a controlled substance is lost in the pharmacy.

14. F, DEA form #222 is used *to order* controlled substances.

15. T

16. T

17. F, When ordering controlled substances, *there is a maximum of 10 different items* that can be ordered on the DEA form.

18. T

19. F, *Schedule V* drugs have no potential for abuse.

20. T

21. T

22. F, The Pure Food and Drug Act of 1906 *did not* include cosmetics.

23. T

24. T

25. T

26. F, *Libel* is defamatory writing.

27. F, *Slander* is spoken words that jeopardize someone's reputation or means of livelihood.

28. T

29. T

30. T

Short Answer

1. See page 61

2. enacted to stop illegal use of drugs; regulates drug trafficking used to support terrorism; legal drugs that can be used in the manufacture of illegal drugs must be kept behind counters or in locked cases; purchases of these drugs must be tracked

3. See page 57

4. See page 55

5. See page 41

Multiple Choice

1. c   2. e   3. a   4. b   5. b   6. a
7. c   8. d   9. d   10. a   11. d

Chapter 4: Pharmaceutical and Medical Terminology and Abbreviations
Matching

Match the term with the definition.

1. D 2. G 3. A 4. B 5. H 6. E
7. C 8. F 9. I

Match the root term to its meaning.

1. E 2. F 3. G 4. B 5. H 6. I
7. D 8. C 9. A 10. J

Match the term with its meaning.

1. X 2. W 3. O 4. V 5. T 6. P 7. U
8. S 9. M 10. R 11. L 12. Q 13. N 14. J
15. I 16. G 17. K 18. F 19. H 20. D 21. E
22. B 23. C 24. A 25. Z 26. Y

True/False

1. T

2. T

3. F: *–itis* is a suffix meaning "inflammation"

4. F: A structure at the beginning of a word that modifies the meaning of the root is a prefix.

5. T

6. F: *Micro-* is a prefix meaning "small"

7. F *Macro-* is a prefix meaning "large"

8. T

9. T

10. T

11. F: Hives are caused by fluid leakage from blood vessels into the layer just beneath the skin's surface.

12. T

13. F: Purpura is purplish discoloration of the skin caused by extravasation of blood into the tissues

14. T

15. T

16. T

17. T

18. T

19. T

20. F: The pharmacy technician should be familiar with medical terminology, abbreviations, and symbols.

Multiple Choice

1. C 2. A 3. C 4. B 5. D 6. D 7. A

Chapter 5: Dosage Forms and Routes of Administration
Matching

Match the term with the definition.

1. D 2. E 3. I 4. A 5. G 6. M 7. B
8. H 9. J 10. K 11. L 12. N 13. O
14. Q 15. R 16. P 17. F 18. U 19. T
20. C 21. S

True/False

1. T

2. T

3. F: New drugs may come from living organisms (organic substances) or nonliving materials (inorganic substances)

4. T

5. F: Certain drugs are soluble in water, some are soluble in alcohol, and others are soluble in a mixture of liquids.

6. F: Most tablets are intended to be swallowed whole for dissolution and absorption from the gastrointestinal tract.

7. F: Buccal tablets are placed between the cheek and the gum until they are dissolved and absorbed.

8. T

9. T

10. F: A hard or semisolid dosage form containing a medication intended for local application in the mouth or throat is called a **troche** or **lozenge.**

11. T

12. T

13. F: Liquid preparations include drugs that have been dissolved or suspended.

14. T

15. T

16. F: At one time, the nicotine transdermal patch was the most popular patch used in the United States.

17. T

18. T

19. T

20. F: The chosen route of drug administration determines the rate and intensity of the drug's effect.

21. T

22. F: Never recap a needle – this will help to avoid needle sticks.

23. T

24. T

25. T

26. T

27. F: Parenteral medications come in vials, ampules, and prefilled syringes.

28. T

Short Answer

1. see page 125

2. see pages 129-132

3. If an intravenous infusion is required for more than 2 to 3 days, a cardiovascular catheter is required.

4. The act of drawing breath, vapor, or gas into the lungs is called inhalation. Inhalation therapy may involve the administration of medicines, water vapor, and gases such as oxygen, carbon dioxide, and helium.

5. see page 129

Multiple Choice

1. B   2. E   3. C   4. A   5. D   6. D
7. A   8. C   9. B   10. D   11. B   12. A
13. B   14. A   15. C

Chapter 6: Overview of Body Systems and Their Functions

Matching

Match the term with the definition.

1. H   2. B   3. F   4. N   5. P   6. S
7. K   8. U   9. Q   10. J   11. I   12. A
13. C   14. V   15. W   16. O   17. M   18. T
19. R   20. G   21. D   22. L   23. E   24. X

True/False

1. T

2. T

3. T

4. F: Certain skin cells called **keratinocytes** assist the immune system.

5. T

6. F: Muscles require electrical impulses from motor nerves for stimulation (see Figure 6-4).

7. T

8. T

9. T

10. T

11. T

12. T

13. F: The nervous system is able to cope with different types of stressors at different times of life, which is part of normal living or mental health.

14. F: The eye is a hollow, spherical structure about 2.5 centimeters in diameter

15. T

16. T

17. F: Frequent or prolonged exposure to sounds with intensities above 85 decibels (dB) can damage the hearing receptors and cause permanent hearing loss.

18. T

19. T

20. F: Endocrine glands secrete hormones, or chemical messengers, directly into the bloodstream.

21. T

22. T

23. T

24. F: The pituitary gland is under the control of the hypothalamus in the brain.

25. T

26. T

27. T

28. F: The adrenal glands are located at the top of each kidney.

29. F: The conversion of glycogen to glucose results in an increase in blood glucose.

30. T

31. T

32. T

33. T

34. T

35. T

36. F: Blood consists of red blood cells, white blood cells, and platelets suspended in a liquid known as *plasma*.

37. T

38. T

39. F: Platelets help to close breaks in blood vessels.

40. T

41. T

42. F: The study of the normal functions of the body.

43. F: The liver is one of the largest organs of the digestive system (see Figure 6-33).

44. T

45. T

Short Answer

1. The nervous system is divided into two sections: the central nervous system (CNS) and the peripheral nervous system (PNS). The central nervous system is located in the dorsal cavity, the brain is enclosed in the cranium, and the spinal cord is inside the spinal cavity. The PNS is outside the CNS and connects the CNS to the remainder of the body. The

2. See page 153

3. See page 153

4. See page 159

5. In medicine, hormones generally are used in three ways: (1) for replacement therapy; (2) for pharmacologic effects beyond replacement; and (3) for endocrine system diagnostic testing.

6. See page 161

Multiple Choice

1. C	2. A	3. D	4. B	5. E	6. A
7. A	8. C	9. C	10. B	11. A	12. D

Chapter 7: Most Common Diseases and Conditions

Matching

Match the term with its definition.

1. A	2. P	3. I	4. Q	5. O	6. K	7. C
8. D	9. J	10. F	11. B	12. L	13. H	
14. G	15. M	16. N	17. E	18. R	19. T	20. S

Match the term to its definition.

1. A	2. C	3. D	4. B	5. E	6. G	7. F
8. H	9. I	10. L	11. K	12. J	13. M	
14. N	15. O					

True/False

1. T

2. F: In the United States, cancer causes more than 500,000 deaths every year

3. T

4. T

5. F: Cardiovascular disorders are the most common causes of death in the United States.

6. T

7. T

8. T

9. T

10. F: The risk of hypertension increases with age, and is higher in African Americans than Caucasians.

11. F: Arrhythmias reduce the efficiency of the heart's pumping cycle.

12. T

13. T

14. T

15. F: Pernicious anemia is characterized by decreased production of hydrochloric acid in the stomach, and a deficiency of **intrinsic factor**, which is normally secreted by the inner layer of the stomach

16. F: Thrombophlebitis is defined as an inflammation inside a vein along with the formation of a blood clot at the site.

17. T

18. T

19. F: Chronic bronchitis is inflammation of the bronchi caused by irritants or infection.

20. T

21. T

22. T

23. T

24. F: Anaphylaxis is an acute, potentially life-threatening type 1 (immediate) hypersensitivity reaction

25. T

26. F: Schizophrenia is a mental illness characterized by distortion of reality, disorganized thought patterns, social withdrawal, hallucinations, and poor judgment. Bipolar disorder is a mental illness characterized by periods of extreme excitation or mania, and deep depression.

27. T

28. T

29. T

30. T

31. T

32. T

33. F: Social anxiety disorder is characterized by an intense, irrational fear of situations in which one might be scrutinized by others, or might do something that is embarrassing or humiliating.

34. F: Insomnia is the inability to fall asleep or stay asleep.

35. T

36. T

37. T

38. F: The development of a cataract is usually slow, causing vision loss and possible blindness if untreated.

39. T

40. T

41. F: A condition of the intestinal tract characterized by patches of inflammation and even ulcers.

42. F: Ulcerative colitis occurs primarily in young adults, especially women

43. T

44. F: The cause of RA has not been established.

45. T

46. T

47. F: Gonorrhea, a common STD, is an infection of the **genitourinary** tract.

48. T

49. T

50. T

Short Answer

1. See page 188

2. See page 189

3. See pages 198 – 203

4. See page 202

5. Macular degeneration

6. See pages 209-210

Multiple Choice

1. D	2. A	3. C	4. E	5. B	6. A	7. D
8. E	9. B	10. B	11. D	12. C	13. E	

Chapter 8: Microbiology
Matching

Match the term to the definition.

1. D	2. A	3. E	4. F	5. H	6. J	7. W
8. G	9. X	10. I	11. B	12. C	13. T	
14. Q	15. K	16. L	17. N	18. U	19. O	
20. V	21. P	22. Y	23. AA	24. EE	25. CC	
26. DD	27. BB	28. Z	29. FF	30. M	31. R	32. S

True/False

1. T

2. T

3. T

4. F: Viruses are organisms that can live only inside cells.

5. T

6. F: Rickettsia are small bacteria incapable of living free of a host

7. T

8. T

9. F: An example is salmonellosis transmitted through contaminated food

10. T

11. T

12. F: Proper handwashing depends on two factors: running water and friction.

13. F: Most microorganisms are beneficial

14. T

15. T

16. F: The two most popular alcohol germicides are ethanol and isopropanol, usually used in 70% to 80% concentrations. Small instruments may be sufficiently disinfected by soaking them in these agents for 10 to 15 minutes.

17. T

18. F: Because they must not destroy too much host tissue, antiseptics are generally not as toxic as disinfectants.

19. T

Multiple Choice

1. C   2. B   3. D   4. A   5. C   6. D   7. D

Short Answer

1. To prevent disease, it is necessary to look at the methods that can be used to minimize the chances of being a carrier of disease. One of the simplest ways of preventing the spread of disease is to practice hand hygiene by washing the hands or using an alcohol-based hand solution.

2. See page 236

3. See page 235

4. See page 235

Chapter 9: Pharmacology
Matching

Match the term to its definition.

1. R	2. Q	3. T	4. S	5. C	6. N
7. K	8. A	9. E	10. F	11. Y	12. D
13. G	14. AA	15. M	16. Z	17. I	18. J
19. V	20. O	21. U	22. P	23. W	24. L
25. B	26. X	27. H			

True/False

1. T

2. T

3. F: Pharmacy technicians need to have a wide understanding of the types of drugs available, as well as their uses. They must understand the action, typical side effects, route of administration, and recommended dose of every medication that may be administered.

4. T

5. F: **Parkinson's disease** is characterized by resting tremor, resistance to passive movement, akinesia (inability to initiate movements), loss of postural reflexes, and behavioral manifestations.

6. F: Depression is one of the most common psychiatric disorders in the United States

7. T

8. T

9. T

10. F: Medications are not the first line of treatment for hyperlipidemia. Antihyperlipidemic drugs are used only if diet modification and exercise programs fail to lower low-density lipoprotein (LDL), or "bad cholesterol" levels, to normal.

11. T

12. T

13. F: Some of the most common disorders in humans at any age are those affecting the musculoskeletal system.

14. T

15. F: Insulin doses are measured in units.

16. T

17. T

18. T

19. F: Vancomycin can destroy most gram-positive organisms.

20. T

21. T

22. T

23. T

24. F: Opioid antidiarrheals are the most effective drugs for controlling diarrhea. Selected

25. T

Multiple Choice

1. A   2. C   3. C   4. D   5. D   6. B   7. C
8. D   9. D   10. C

Short Answer

1. See page 254

2. See page 257-258

3. See page 272-273

4. A reaction, referred to as Red Man Syndrome, may occur if the drug is given too rapidly. Flushing and/or a rash affecting the face, neck, and upper torso characterize this syndrome. It may also cause hypotension and angioedema (rapid swelling of the skin, mucosa, and submucosal tissues).

5. See TABLE 9-9 and TABLE 9-10 on page 238

6. See TABLE 9-12 on page 259

Chapter 10: Immunology and Vaccines

Matching

Match the term with its definition.

1. J	2. O	3. L	4. A	5. D	6. M
7. F	8. R	9. C	10. Q	11. I	12. N
13. P	14. B	15. H	16. K	17. G	18. E

Match the term to its definition.

1. B	2. E	3. P	4. J	5. M	6. O
7. A	8. D	9. K	10. C	11. G	12. I
13. N	14. H	15. L	16. F		

Match the term to its definition.

1. E	2. A	3. B	4. D	5. C	6. J
7. I	8. H	9. G	10. F	11. K	12. N
13. M	14. L	15. O			

True/False

1. T

2. T

3. F: A person who is susceptible to a disease usually has inadequate levels of protective antibodies or insufficient nonspecific defenses.

4. T

5. F: Vaccines made from living organisms are the most effective

6. T

7. F: In some states, pharmacists are allowed to administer selected immunizations, such as flu vaccines, in retail (community) pharmacies.

8. T

9. T

10. F: Adverse reactions include local or severe systemic reactions.

11. F: Mumps is an acute viral illness.

12. T

13. T

14. T

15. F: Anthrax was first used effectively as a bioterrorist agent in 2001

Multiple Choice

1. D	2. B	3. A	4. B	5. C	6. D	7. B

Short Answer

1. First Line: Physical barriers, such as the skin and mucous membranes, and chemical barriers that prevent pathogen entry. Second line: Nonspecific defensive cells (eosinophils, phagocytes, natural killer cells) and proteins. Third line: Immune system, which has specific targets and memory.

2. See pages 306-307

3. See page 315

4. See page 314

5. See pages 295-296

Chapter 11: Nutrition

1. CC	2. Y	3. Z	4. V	5. X	6. BB
7. W	8. AA	9. DD	10. E	11. U	12. D
13. K	14. I	15. H	16. G	17. F	18. J
19. Q	20. P	21. O	22. N	23. M	24. L
25. R	26. S	27. T	28. B	29. A	30. C

True/False

1. T

2. F: A water-soluble substance that is the common pharmaceutical form of vitamin B_{12}.

3. T

4. F: **High-density lipoproteins (HDLs)** are Lipoproteins that carry cholesterol from cells to the liver for eventual excretion. **Low-density lipoproteins (LDLs)** are Lipoproteins that carry blood cholesterol from all cells. **Very low-density lipoproteins (VLDLs)** are Lipoproteins made by the liver to transport lipids throughout the body.

5. T

6. T

7. T

8. T

9. F: **Sodium** (Na) is one of the most important elements in the body

10. T

11. T

12. F: Human growth and development require both nutritional and psychosocial support.

13. F: Protein is the major source of building material for muscles, blood, skin, hair, nails, and the internal organs.

14. T

15. T

16. T

17. T

18. F: Exposure to the sun for 10 minutes every day allows your skin to provide enough vitamin D for your body.

19. F: Natural vitamin K is stored in the body and is not toxic

20. T

21. T

22. T

23. T

24. T

25. F: Pharmacy technicians must be familiar with basic nutrition dietary standards and pathological conditions. In pharmacy practice, there are many questions that clients may ask about foods and nutrition.

Multiple Choice

1. B   2. A   3. D   4. A   5. C   6. B   7. B
8. A   9. D   10. D

Short Answer

1. **Hypervitaminosis** - An abnormal condition resulting from excessive intake of toxic amounts of one or more vitamins, especially over a long period. **Hypovitaminosis** - A condition related to the deficiency of one or more vitamins.

2. See pages 339-340

3. See pages 336-337

4. See TABLE 11-4 on page 343

Chapter 12: Food and Drug Interactions
Matching

Match the term to its definition.

1. B   2. E   3. D   4. A   5. C

True/False

1. F: Some drug-related problems develop unexpectedly, without being predicted.

2. T

3. T

4. T

5. F: Many drug-related problems are caused by drug interaction. Pharmacy technicians must be familiar with this important matter and understand factors that may have an effect on different agents.

6. F: Sometimes an individual may see more than one physician or two or more specialists in addition to a family physician. Thus, it is difficult for any one of these physicians to be aware of all the drugs that have been prescribed by the others for this patient.

7. T

8. F: Newborn infants do not have fully developed enzyme systems.

9. T

10. T

11. T

12. T

13. F: Chronic use of alcoholic beverages may increase the rate of metabolism of drugs such as warfarin, phenytoin, and tolbutamide, probably by increasing the activity of liver enzymes.

14. T

15. F: Maintaining complete and current medication records for patients is essential.

16. T

17. T

18. T

19. F: Promethazine is the generic name for Phenergan®

20. T

Multiple Choice

1. B   2. A   3. D   4. A   5. C

Short Answer

1. See pages 358-359

2. Age, Genetic Factors, Diseases and Conditions of Patients, Diet, Alcohol Consumption, Smoking

3. Diazepam, Theophylline, Chlorpromazine, and Amitriptyline

Chapter 13: Medication Errors

1. I   2. A   3. B   4. H   5. G   6. F   7. E
8. D   9. C

True/False

1. T

2. T

3. F: Highly trained people still make mistakes. Even if clinicians are well-educated and follow policies, procedures, or other guidelines, errors will still happen.

4. T

5. F: Never assume that a patient is the correct person to receive a medication without verifying his or her name.

6. F: Dosing errors are the most common medication errors that occur in adults and children.

7. T

8. T

9. T

10. T

11. F: Stress is often linked to a variety of outcomes, and certainly plays a part in medication errors.

12. F: Every patient's pain tolerance level is different.

13. F: Patients should be encouraged to ask questions about their medications.

14. T

15. T

16. F: Pharmacists and technicians can join an electronic mailing list to get up-to-date information that the FDA disseminates.

17. T

18. F: Labels should be checked and compared with physicians' orders at least three times to ensure accuracy.

19. T

20. T

Multiple Choice

1. B   2. C   3. D   4. D   5. C   6. A   7. D
8. C   9. B

Short Answer

1. See pages 374-376

2. Confirm patient's identity, Verify original prescription, Verify medication calculation, Communicate concerns to the pharmacist, Verify patient allergy history, Inquire if patient has questions for pharmacist, Maintain continuing education

3. See page 384

Chapter 14: Basic Mathematics

1. D   2. O   3. J   4. K   5. G   6. S   7. L
8. Q   9. E   10. M   11. P   12. B   13. I
14. U   15. F   16. T   17. C   18. R   19. H
20. A   21. N

True/False

1. T

2. F: Roman numerals are used less commonly than Arabic numbers in dosage calculation.

3. T

4. T

5. T

6. T

7. T

8. T

9. T

10. T

Problem Solving

1. Q6h = every 6 hours which means $24 \div 6 = 4$ doses in 24 hours

$$4 \times 10 \text{ mg} = 40 \text{ mg}$$

$$\frac{15 \text{ mg}}{1 \text{ ml}} = \frac{40 \text{ mg}}{X}$$

$$\frac{15 X}{15} = \frac{40}{15}$$

$$X = 2.67 \text{ ml}$$

2. Make any necessary conversions (concentrations are measured in mg/ml)

1 gram = 1000 mg

$$\frac{1000 \text{ mg Vancomycin}}{20 \text{ ml}} = \frac{X \text{ mg}}{1 \text{ ml}}$$

cross multiply and solve for X

20 X = 1000

X = 50 mg/ml

3. 4 ml

$$\frac{2.5 \text{ mg}}{1 \text{ ml}} = \frac{10 \text{ mg}}{X}$$

$$2.5 \times (X) = 10 \times 1$$

$$\frac{2.5 X}{2.5} = \frac{10}{2.5}$$

X = 4 ml

4. 20 ml

$$\frac{20 \text{ mEq}}{10 \text{ ml}} = \frac{2 \text{ mEq}}{1 \text{ ml}}$$
Reduce 20mEq per 10ml to 2mEq/ml

$$\frac{40 \text{ mEq}}{X} = \frac{2 \text{ mEq}}{1 \text{ ml}}$$

$$40 \times 1 = 2X$$

$$\frac{40}{2} = \frac{2X}{2}$$

20 ml = X

5.

Chapter 15: Measurement Systems

Matching

Match the term with its definition.

1. L   2. K   3. J   4. I   5. M   6. H   7. A
8. E   9. F   10. G   11. D   12. C   13. B

True/False

1. T

2. T

3. F, One liter is equal to 1000 milliliters.

4. T

5. F: 1 lb equals 453.59 g.

6. T

7. F: Household measurements are not accurate enough for health care professionals to use in the calculation of drug dosages in the hospital or pharmacy.

8. F: 240 mL is equal to 8 oz.

9. T

10. T

11. T

12. F: There are 2 tablespoons in one ounce

13. T

14. T

15. T

Multiple Choice

1. A   2. C   3. B   4. C   5. C

Short Answer

1. Three systems are used for measuring medication and solutions: **metric system**, **apothecary system**, and **household system**.

2. 215.6 lbs.

3. 113.64 kg.

Unit Conversions

1. 0.5 g	2. 88 lbs	3. 4 L
4. 8 oz	5. 1,000,000 mg	6. 0.35 mg
7. 45,450 mL	8. 120 mg	9. 0.1 mg
10. 0.6 kg	11. 240 mL	12. 1.08 gr
13. 0.025 g	14. 45 mL	15. 1500 mg

16. 1 kg   17. 500 mg   18. 7.5 gr
19. 93.5 in   20. 0.008 L   21. 10,000 mcg
22. 0.004 g   23. 0.3 kg   24. 2 cups
25. 2.03 cups   26. 473.176 mL   27. 32 oz
28. 48 t   29. 29.6 mL   30. 0.006 kg
31. 68.04 kg   32. 2 T

Problem Solving

1. 12 tablets per day; 3 10 mg tablets 4 times per day

2. 15 tablets; ½ tablet 3 times a day

3. 21 tablets; 1 ½ tablets twice a day

4. 2 tablets each morning

Chapter 16: Calculation of Dosages

1. C   2. F   3. G   4. H   5. A   6. I   7. B
8. E   9. D

True/False

1. T

2. T

3. F: To prevent medication errors, the technician should remember the following: right patient, right route, right drug, right technique, right dose, right documentation, right time

4. F: The NDC number is a unique identifying number that every prescription medication must have.

5. T

6. T

7. T

8. T

9. F: When a liquid medication is measured, hold the transparent measuring device at eye level.

10. T

11. T

12. F: Heparin is a potent anticoagulant that prevents clot formation and blood coagulation.

13. F: Heparin can be administered IV or SC.

14. T

15. F: To measure the flow rate, the drip chamber must be squeezed until it is half full, making it easier to appropriately count the number of drops falling into the chamber.

16. F: Macrodrop tubing is used for fluids infused at a higher rate, for example, infusions that are set at 80 mL/hr or higher. Microdrop tubing is used for slower infusions for which accuracy of dosage delivery is essential, such as in critical care or pediatric settings.

17. T

18. T

Multiple Choice

1. D   2. A   3. C   4. D   5. C   6. B

Short Answer

1. See page 437

2. See page 439-442

3. See page 463

4. See page 464-465

Problem Solving

1. 2.88 mL

2. 20 mL per dose

3. 10 mL per dose

4. 6.67 mL per dose

5. 8 days

6. 625 mL

7. 10 mL would provide a 0.5-mg dose; the multiple dose vial would provide 150 doses

8. 0.18 grams

9.
- 2.09 mL
- 28 doses
- approximately 15 days
- 9,520 mcg
- 125.4 mL

10.
- 798 mg
- 40 mL
- 16.7 grams
- 6 doses
- 2 days
- 838 mL

11.

- 330 mg

- 6.6 mL

- 13.2 grams

- 27 doses

- 6.8 days (roughly, 6 full days and 3 out of the 4 doses on the 7th day)

- 264 mL

12. 16.67 gtt / min

13. 50 gtt / min

14. 50 mL / hour

15.

- 93.7 mL / hour

- 93.7 gtt / min

16. 5 hours

Chapter 17: Safety in the Workplace

1. J   2. K   3. I   4. H   5. G   6. F   7. E
8. D   9. C   10. A   11. B

True/False

1. F: OSHA establishes safety regulations for employers and monitors compliance.

2. T

3. T

4. F: The top diamond is red and indicates a flammability hazard.

5. T

6. T

7. T

8. F: OSHA regulations require that all healthcare workers be immunized against hepatitis B, because they are at risk for exposure to blood-borne pathogens.

9. F: Companies with more than 10 employees must maintain records of all work-related injuries and illnesses.

10. T

11. F: Any materials that have come into contact with blood or body fluids are treated as hazardous waste. Various containers are used to collect hazardous material. Waste containers are labeled with the **biohazard symbol** to ensure that all employees are aware of the contents (see Figure 17-6). Plastic bags are used for gloves, paper towels, dressings, and other soft material; rigid containers are used for sharps such as needles, glass slides, scalpel blades, or disposable syringes.

12. T

13. T

14. T

15. T

16. T

17. T

Multiple Choice

1. B   2. A   3. B   4. D   5. D

Short Answer

1. See pages 475–476

2. See page 476

3. See page 480

Chapter 18: Hospital Pharmacy Practice

Matching

Match the term with its definition.

1. G   2. H   3. L   4. N   5. M   6. O   7. K
8. F   9. E   10. D   11. C   12. B   13. A   14. I
15. J   16. P   17. Y   18. X   19. W   20. V
21. U   22. T   23. S   24. R   25. Q

Match the organization with its mission.

1. C   2. A   3. D   4. E   5. B

True/False

1. F: Dispensing processes have become much more sophisticated than in the past in response to the need to handle a variety of different types of medication orders.

2. T

3. T

4. F: The director of pharmacy is responsible for maintaining an adequate medication inventory and establishing specifications for the

procurement of all drugs, chemicals, and biologic agents related to the practice of pharmacy.

5. F: The medication fulfillment process begins in the pharmacy department when a copy of the original medication order is received in the department.

6. F: The role of the pharmacist has changed from being a product dispenser to having expanding responsibility for the entire medication process.

7. T

8. T

9. T

10. F: Human intervention can never be replaced.

11. T

12. F: Pharmacy technicians must always utilize aseptic technique when preparing products of contamination.

13. T

14. T

15. T

16. F: The label should also contain the initials of the person dispensing the drug.

17. T

Multiple Choice

1. B   2. E   3. C   4. B   5. E   6. A   7. D
8. B

Short Answer

1. See page 496

2. See page 497

3. See page 506

Chapter 19: Community Pharmacy
Matching

Match the term with its definition.

1. F   2. A   3. G   4. H   5. I   6. E   7. D
8. C   9. B

True/False

1. T

2. T

3. T

4. T

5. F: It is a legal requirement that the prescription order be numbered and that the same number be placed on the label.

6. T

7. F: Auxiliary labels (also known as strip labels) are used to emphasize important aspects of the dispensed medication, including its proper use, handling, storage, refill status, and necessary warnings or precautions

8. F: To prevent contamination of capsules and tablets, the counting tray should be wiped clean after each use, because powder, especially from uncoated tablets, tends to remain on the tray.

9. T

10. T

11. F: A prescription for a controlled substance (Schedules II through V) must be handled carefully. The lower the number of the drug schedule, the higher the potential for abuse of the drug

12. T

13. T

14. T

15. T

16. T

Multiple Choice

1. C   2. B   3. C   4. C   5. A   6. D   7. D

Short Answer

1. See page 527

2. See page 531

3. See page 539-540

Chapter 20: Advanced Pharmacy
Matching

Match the term with the definition.

1. G   2. F   3. E   4. D   5. N   6. M   7. I
8. H   9. L   10. K   11. J   12. V   13. U   14. T
15. S   16. R   17. Q   18. P   19. O   20. B   21. C
22. A

True/False

1. T

2. F: There are now more long-term facility beds than acute care beds.

3. T

4. T

5. F: Home infusion pharmacy is a sterile compounding practice that is similar (but not identical) to a hospital pharmacy practice.

6. T

7. F: A hospice pharmacy can be part of a traditional community pharmacy, in which hospice is a part of its business, or it can be a pharmacy that services only hospice patients.

8. T

9. T

10. F: Central fill pharmacies reduce costs, provide patients with more options concerning their prescriptions, and allow local pharmacists at individual pharmacies to have more time for patient counseling.

11. T

12. T

13. T

14. T

15. T

Multiple Choice

1. A 2. D 3. D 4. B 5. D

Short Answer

1. See page 553

2. See page 555

3. See page 561

4. See page 561

Chapter 21: Extemporaneous Prescription Compounding
Matching

Match the term to its definition.

1. I 2. E 3. L 4. O 5. G 6. S 7. N
8. H 9. K 10. F 11. A 12. M 13. B 14. R
15. C 16. T 17. Q 18. D 19. P 20. J

True/False

1. T

2. T

3. T

4. F: Spatulas are available in stainless steel, plastic, or hard rubber. They must be clean and have indented edges.

5. T

6. T

7. T

8. F: Quality control and proper documentation of all products are essential.

9. T

10. T

Multiple Choice

1. D 2. A 3. D 4. C 5. E

Short Answer

1. See page 595

2. Preparation of sterile products requires special skills and training. Sterile products must be prepared in a clean room, using aseptic technique (discussed in Chapter 22). Dry powders of parenteral drugs for reconstitution are used for drug products that are unstable as solutions. It is important to know the correct diluents that can be used to yield a solution

3. The pharmacy technician must be trained and skilled to compound medication under the supervision of the pharmacist.

4. The extemporaneous compounding of sterile products is no longer confined only to the hospital environment. It is now done by community pharmacists engaged in home care practice. Quality control and proper documentation of all products are essential. Preparation of sterile products requires special skills and training.

5. See page 595

Chapter 22: Sterile Compounding
Matching

Match the term with its definition.

1. E 2. D 3. C 4. B 5. A 6. F 7. G
8. H 9. M 10. N 11. L 12. K 13. J 14. I

True/False

1. T

2. T

3. F: Parenteral products should be isotonic; the correct level of isotonicity depends on the route of administration

4. F: Parenteral products must be chemically, physically, and microbiologically stable

5. T

6. T

7. F: Proper hand washing depends on two factors: running water and friction. The water should be warm, because water that is too cold or too hot will cause the skin to become chapped. Friction involves the firm rubbing of all surfaces of the hands and wrists.

8. T

9. F: Living tissue surfaces such as skin cannot be sterilized, but can be rendered as free of pathogens as possible with the use of a sterile covering.

10. T

11. F: Gas sterilization is commonly used in hospitals that have room-sized gas sterilization chambers.

12. T

13. T

14. T

15. T

16. F: The air moves at a rate of 90 to 120 linear feet per minute, with very little turbulence, at a uniform velocity.

17. T

18. T

19. T

20. T

21. F: The process for compounding ophthalmics properly takes from 1 to 2 weeks.

Multiple Choice

1. D   2. B   3. C   4. D   5. A   6. C   7. B

Short Answer

1. See page 603

2. See pages 603-607

3. See pages 608-611

4. See page 612

5. Pharmacokinetics – Rates of absorption for any routes of administration besides intravenous or intra-arterial, rates of distribution, rates of metabolism, and rates of excretion will have an effect on the selected route of administration and type of formulation

6. See pages 616-617

Chapter 23: Management of Pharmacy Operations
Matching

Match the term with its definition.

1. J   2. I   3. H   4. G   5. F   6. E   7. D
8. C   9. B   10. L   11. M   12. K   13. A

True/False

1. F: Pharmacy practice has changed dramatically over the last several years.

2. F: The need for pharmacy managers has increased.

3. T

4. T

5. T

6. F: Indirect costs relate to morbidity and mortality (including illness, disability, and death).

7. T

8. T

9. F: Colored or dated price stickers are another simple and effective manual technique used for ordering.

10. T

11. T

12. T

13. T

14. F: Files may be kept as hard copy (on paper) or on the computer disk.

15. T

16. T

17. T

18. T

19. T

20. F: Expired compounded or repackaged pharmaceuticals cannot be returned and must be disposed of.

21. T

Multiple Choice

1. D   2. B   3. D   4. A   5. A

Short Answer

1. See pages 631-632

2. See page 632

3. See pages 635-636

4. Drug packages must have four basic functions:

   1. Protect their contents from deleterious environmental effects.

   2. Protect their contents from deterioration resulting from handling.

   3. Identify their contents completely and precisely.

   4. Permit their contents to be used quickly, easily, and safely.

Chapter 24: Health Insurance
Matching

Match the term with its definition.

1. N	2. M	3. L	4. K	5. Q	6. P	7. O
8. R	9. S	10. T	11. F	12. E	13. D	14. C
15. B	16. A	17. G	18. H	20. I		

True/False

1. T

2. F: The higher the deductible is, the lower the cost of the policy and the lower the deductible is, the higher the cost of the policy.

3. T

4. T

5. F: Pharmacy technicians must be familiar with many different aspects of health insurance billing and transactions.

6. T

7. T

8. F: Time limitations are set forth for the prompt reporting of workers' compensation cases.

9. T

10. F: **Medicare** is the largest single medical benefits program in the United States

11. T

12. F: Patients (in certain states) who are eligible for Medicare Part B *and* Medicaid may have their monthly Medicare Part B premiums paid for by Medicaid.

13. T

14. F: When you first become eligible for Medicare, you may choose to join or not join into Part D

15. T

16. T

17. T

18. T

19. F: Most of these outstanding amounts are paid within 30 to 60 days after the date of service.

20. T

Multiple Choice

1. B   2. C   3. D   4. A   5. B

Short Answer

1. See page 644

2. See pages 645-646

3. See page 648

4. See page 652

5. See page 653

Chapter 25: Documentation, Billing, and Collection
Matching

Match the term with its definition.

| 1. D | 2. M | 3. L | 4. K | 5. J | 6. H | 7. C |
| 8. A | 9. G | 10. F | 11. E | 12. B | 13. I | |

True/False

1. F: Documentation of all pharmacy activities is very important,

2. T

3. F: Electronic billing has become the industry standard, with paper forms greatly reduced in today's pharmacy. Documentation is actually made easier

by electronic billing and reimbursement activities because the storage of this information is more easily referenced and located.

4. T

5. T

6. T

7. F: Federal and state laws require all personnel, including pharmacy technicians, to help manage controlled substances located in the workplace.

8. F: It is also important to ensure confidentiality requirements and at the same time maximize retrieval speed.

9. T

10. F: The hospital pharmacy differs from the retail or community pharmacy in various ways.

11. T

12. F: The staff of the hospital pharmacy have little interaction with patients concerning billing and collections.

13. T

14. T

15. F: Pharmacy technicians are responsible for documenting billing and reimbursement activities correctly in case of future audits.

Multiple Choice

1. D   2. B   3. A   4. B

Short Answer

1. See page 664

2. See page 665

3. See page 669

Chapter 26: Inventory Control
Matching

Match the term with its definition.

1. C   2. G   3. F   4. A   5. E   6. D   7. B

True/False

1. F: Proper inventory control systems help to streamline the hectic activities of the pharmacies of today

2. T

3. T

4. T

5. F: Inventory turnover rate = Purchases over a period of time divided by the average inventory for the period

6. F: The "lead time" is assumed to be zero, as orders to replenish stock are made when the inventory level reduces to zero or another pre-determined "critical" level.

7. T

8. T

9. T

10. F: The state board of pharmacy could start an investigation if financial statements seem incorrect or possibly suspect.

11. T

12. T

13. T

14. F: Automated dispensing systems are becoming the normal way of dispensing in many pharmacy settings.

15. F: Most automated dispensing systems comply with the regulations of both the Health Insurance Portability and Accountability Act and the Joint Commission

16. T

17. T

18. F: Automation in the pharmacy is becoming the wave of the future, with many dispensing functions being handled by robotic machinery.

19. T

20. T

Multiple Choice

1. D   2. D   3. A   4. D   5. A

Short Answer

1. See pages 678- 682

2. See page 683

3. See pages 678-682

Chapter 27: Computers in the Pharmacy

Matching

Match the term with its definition.

1. F	2. N	3. M	4. H	5. G	6. L	7. J
8. D	9. K	10. I	11. C	12. B	13. A	14. E

True/False

1. T

2. F: If computers are used properly, then they can significantly decrease the cost of any operation that involves the processing of information;

3. T

4. F: The CPU is the "brains" of the computer.

5. T

6. T

7. T

8. F: Displays use tiny dots of light called "pixels" to make up the various graphical components on their screens.

9. T

10. T

11. T

12. F: Laser printers are preferred over inkjet and other types of printers because of their speed, precision, and economy.

13. T

14. T

15. T

16. T

17. T

18. F: PDAs are usually not much larger than the user's palm and resemble hand-held video games (see Figure 27-6).

19. T

20. T

21. T

Multiple Choice

1. D   2. B   3. A   4. D   5. C

Short Answer

1. See page 701

2. See page 702

3. See pages 707-708

4. See page 711

Chapter 28: Communications

1. R	2. G	3. V	4. M	5. P	6. F	7. N
8. T	9. C	10. U	11. J	12. W	13. H	14. S
15. D	16. L	17. E	18. A	19. K	20. B	
21. Q	22. O	23. I				

Match the term with its meaning

1. C   2. E   3. A   4. D   5. B

True/False

1. T

2. T

3. T

4. F: Proper diction and enunciation are required for speaking clearly and accurately

5. F: Verbal communication consists of much more than just words. Tone, inflection, and level of pitch determine the meaning of the message we are sending even more than the words we choose.

6. F: It is essential that pharmacy technicians are able to communicate effectively with patients, their caregivers, and other health care providers

7. T

8. T

9. F: In a pharmacy, customers are not only clients with a prescription. Customers are also the physicians who write the prescriptions, the nurses who call in the prescriptions, and others, such as pharmaceutical representatives.

10.T

Fill in the Blank

1. understanding

2. tone, inflection

3. written

4. nonverbal

5. open, closed

Multiple Choice

1. C   2. D   3. C   4. D   5. B   6. D